The Unleashed Human

The Ultimate Guide
To Unchain Yourself From Eczema

Dr. TJ Woodham

DEDICATION

This book is dedicated to:
Paul A. Goldberg, MPH, DC, DACBN, DCBCN
and
David Tener, BS, DC

Through their guidance, my health, my life and my skin will never be the same.
My gratitude cannot be explained through words alone. It is time to pay it forward to you and the world.

You can find Dr. Goldberg and Dr. Tener at:
The Goldberg Clinic For Chronic Disease Reversal in Marietta, GA

Furthermore:
I want to express my utmost gratitude to my dear friend Geoffrey Fredd who was a major player in allowing me to create this platform for you. He believed in my message and allowed me to serve you to the highest level possible. All my thanks and love for you Geoff.

Contents

What This Book Is About and What It Is Not About

Hey there, my name is Dr. TJ Woodham….
Before we get started, I want to introduce myself and let you know what this book is about and more importantly, what it is not about.

This book is **NOT** about how to clear your Eczema in a day or week – yet I'm going to show you exactly how to clear your skin in a very short amount of time and have it look better than ever before.

This book is **NOT** another fad diet or cookie cutter approach to better skin and health – yet I will teach you the core principals of eating the correct foods and adopting the lifestyle approaches that will never become obsolete.

This is book is **NOT** just about better skin – yet you will find that along with your skin clearing up COMPLETELY, you will notice a myriad of other incredible health benefits you may not have realized The Unleashed Human lifestyle would give you.

If you have been struggling with chronic eczema for a while now, you may think that your issue lies on the surface of your skin. You have been applying all the natural ointments, balms, concoctions, lotions, soaps to alleviate your poor skin, right? You have also been to the dermatologist and my guess is that you were sent home with a tube of corticosteroids for "atopic dermatitis," which literally translates to Inflammation on the top of your skin. Big word with very little meaning.

I want to let you know, it's not your fault for being misinformed and misguided by the medical community. It is also not the medical community's fault for giving you these protocols, as this is their standard of care. It is what they are taught in medical school and it is how they know how to treat conditions.

The saying "beauty is more than skin deep" has been used to depict how we should accept the personality of a human being before we judge their physical appearance. Yes, we all know this.

The saying "beauty is more than skin deep" has been used to explain how we should first accept someone for their personality before we judge them by their physical appearance. Yes, we all know this. However, this quote has another meaning for Eczema sufferers. The reason why you haven't been set free of your dry, itchy, oozing, scaly skin is because IT ISNT COMING FROM YOUR SKIN.

Health comes from the inside of your body and presents itself on your SKIN! Have you ever noticed how your face and skin look after a night of no sleep or after drinking a good amount of alcohol? It doesn't look pretty right? You will have dark bags under your eyes and your face will look puffy. This is a direct response from the massive amount stress you placed on your liver, your blood stream, your adrenal glands and your immune system.

Can you see how you treat your insides has a direct affect and correlation as to how your skin will look? It is not only the consumption of foods and drinks, but the environment we live in has a big role in your healing. This will be covered in detail later.

I hope that made sense to you. If not, don't stress. This book provides a lot of value and knowledge that will create an awakening for your life. You will read things you have never heard before anywhere and that's okay! I'm super excited to share it with you! Take your time and enjoy the process. You WILL get through this. Even if you have no support system or someone to lean on, you should know that I believe in you ☺.
                              YOU GOT THIS!

For more info, join our Exclusive Facebook group for goodies:
The Unleashed Human

The Start of Your Beautiful Life

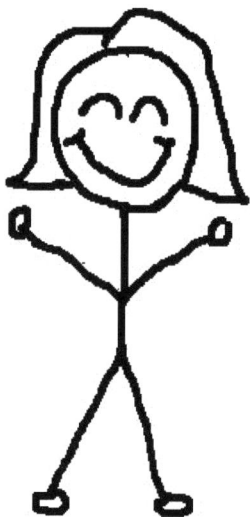

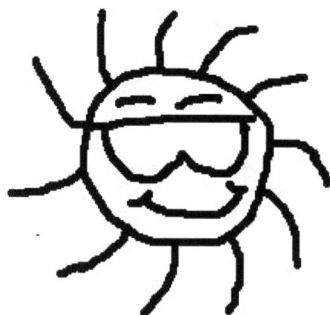

"Life is really simple, but we insist on making it difficult."
-Confucius

Please let me be the first to say CONGRATULATIONS for taking your first MASSIVE step towards incredible skin and super human health! I know for most of you it has been a super long and uphill battle to defeat eczema. If you are here reading this, it means you are a super determined and strong-willed human being. It means that you never settle for anything but AMAZING. It means that you want to be a shining representation of what it truly means to be healthy. It means you want to be a role model for your peers, family and friends. It means that no matter how hard the journey has been for you, the struggle will always be worth it to get your ultimate result: ECZEMA FREE! Your struggle and your story DEFINE YOUR LIFE.

Nobody will ever be able to take this away from you. Realize that your uniqueness separates you from the crowd. Although human nature has tendency to feel embarrassment by being different, you should celebrate moments of pure singularity. Think of it this way: you are a one-man wolf-pack. You are on your own in the wild and you are on a mission. You are the ruler of one and the servant of none. You make your own decisions and create your own life experiences. Choose a life that is guided by your own ability to create moments of happiness, not embarrassment. The human mind makes up whatever you tell it to believe. Our brains are hardwired to think worst case scenario. It is your job to re-frame all negativity and learn to live with your present time.

In this book, I will tell and show you EXACTLY how I defeated eczema and how you can too! I will finally reveal what took me from a mutant, to a superhuman.

Let me ask you a few questions. Michelangelo didn't paint the Sistine Chapel overnight did he? Arnold Schwarzenegger didn't grow massive biceps and triceps by working out one time in the gym, right? Tony Robbins didn't captivate an audience of One Billion by just giving one talk to an audience of 9,000, right? The process of TRUE healing won't be an overnight success as most humans wish it could be. Sorry, but it doesn't work that way. Sure, you can continue to bank on the latest magic potion or drug but sadly it will cost you THOUSANDS of dollars and time spent without any result.

I will admit that that it was certainly a long road to finally come to my wits. I went through years of putting steroid cream all over my body. Years of trying to find every concoction possible to alleviate my eczema, and guess what? None of it actually did anything. The approaches I took either made my eczema worse or put a temporary band aid over all of the symptoms I was experiencing. Each attempt of defeating eczema set me back even further and in turn, made my health worse. I also lost a good amount of money and sanity while in the process.

The crazy thing is that the answer was always there waiting for me. The process I take you through will be challenging. A life without challenge is a life unlived. If you follow me through every step of the way, your results will speak for itself. It certainly takes a focused attitude and mind of determination. The biggest motivator must always be the end goal in mind. Your greatest desire is to finally crush eczema, correct? You must imagine a world where you are eczema free and your skin is glowing. Imagine how incredibly invigorating and liberating that must feel. Always keep this at the forefront of your dreams and desires. You've already made an incredible leap forward by purchasing this book. From here, the only thing I see for your future is true health, happiness and confidence to show the world how POWERFUL you are.

This book covers a wide gambit of habits that the general population fails to take into consideration. These habits, however, yield monumental results. We cover categories ranging from nutrition, sleep habits, and even sunlight exposure times. It is the routine, commitment and repetition that will set you over the top to attain an impenetrable mind and healthy digestive tract. You might feel the urge to skip ahead in chapters, and that is okay. Just know, that when it comes time to implement these routines, they should be done in order. Each habit I show you complements the one before it and the one after it.

Do not feel like you must jump into this immediately. The last thing I want you to feel is overwhelmed. Take your time! Go at your own pace. I don't want you to quit because it was too much at first. You may need to take baby steps and that is okay! Everyone has their own speed. Just know that when you get to where you need to be, your eczema will be yesterday's problem.

The intention of this book is to give you tremendous value, while also making it easy to read. This book was designed for anyone to pick up and implement easy concepts that may seem like miniscule lifestyle modifications but make a world of difference. This book is short and to the point. It was not my intention to fill you with a bunch of facts but rather give you actionable steps to crush eczema. I also intend to provide valuable education that you were never taught growing up. There is a lot of extra content that complements the many modifications I provide. If you understand the WHY of the lifestyle modifications, it will make much more sense on the HOW and WHAT.

I do not want this to be categorized as a new fad diet approach because it's not. This is evergreen. This lifestyle approach will never age. It will remain relevant 1,000 years from now.

I know how many times I searched to find the answer to my eczema and how many times I came up empty handed. If you follow me, this will be your last stop on this wild train. This is your final destination. This is where you finally become an unleashed human.

Break the chains.

You've been reborn.

The Story That Gave Me Power

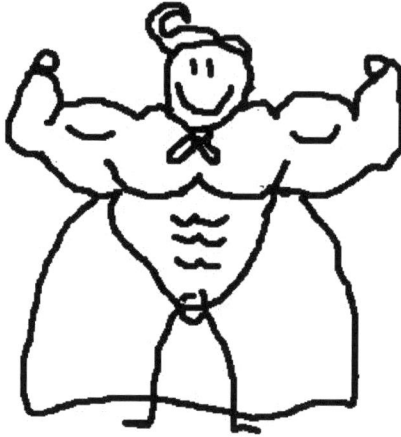

"The past cannot change. The future is yet in your power."
-Unknown

It was summer 2013 and I was at the University of Florida as a Biology major. It was my senior year and I noticed that my skin started to become inflamed with red splotches. I thought nothing of it until it seemed to spread to other parts of my body. It had even spread to my private parts. It was at this point that I needed to see a dermatologist. Upon visiting the dermatologist, I remember waiting in the cold exam room and I heard many voices approaching the door. I initially thought I would just be seeing the attending doctor. Boy was I wrong. In walked not only the female doctor, but FIVE other female interns. There I was completely exposed for all 6 women to see my private parts in an embarrassing state of health. What an experience huh?

After this excellent life experience, it was no surprise that the dermatologist very lazily diagnosed my Eczema as "atopic dermatitis", which literally translates into "inflammation of the skin." It amazes me that many medical doctors go through six to eight years of medical schooling and these are the kind of diagnoses they give people. While also giving EVERY person a prescription for corticosteroid cream. GREAT. Good thing these drugs DON'T DO ANYTIHNG but place a temporary band aid over a more serious underlying condition.

At the time, being young and naive, I still trusted in western medicine approach to health care, so I continued to follow the plan of care. I used the steroid cream for a good couple of months to no avail. The eczema returned. At the time, having no knowledge of the power of the CORRECT food, ADEQUATE sunlight and stress MANAGEMENT, I would continue the process of bodily harm.

Fall 2013, I was volunteering and doing research in the University of Florida's dental school. I was on track for a 2014 admittance into UF's dental program. It wasn't until my good friend from high school reached out to me and advised me to look into the Chiropractic profession. My friend, knowing that I always had a passion for human performance, manual therapies, and nutrition, thought it would be a better route than smelling breath for the rest of my life.

Before deciding the fate of my career, I learned that Chiropractors not only undergo EXTENSIVE education about the bio-mechanics human spine, but also undertake HUNDREDS of hours in TRUE Clinical Nutrition. I read incredible stories of people getting rid of diseases that were deemed "incurable" by the medical community. Diseases like ulcerative colitis, Crohn's, IBS, rheumatoid arthritis, you name it, chiropractors were getting rid of them.

Putting on my skeptic hat, I dug deeper as to how they were doing it. It wasn't rocket science. They were simply providing the right environment and nutrients for a human being to thrive. It all made sense from then on. I knew this was my calling. It wasn't easy making such a massive change in direction, considering I also had much backlash from family and friends. However, I decided to take a leap of faith to apply to Life University Chiropractic College and never look back.

Now during my transition from UF to Life University, I was very much into working out. Let's just say I WAS A MEATHEAD. I WAS A GYM BULLY. ALL I CARED ABOUT WAS LIFTING. Don't get me wrong, they were some of the best times of my life. I crushed personal records and loved being one of the strongest guys in the gym, but my health and self-relationships were suffering for it. I was working out seven days a week, with my "rest" day being comprised of sprints and dead lifts. I weighed 180 pounds at 5'10 with 6% body fat. I was squatting 405 pounds, chest pressing 130-pound dumbbells in each arm for 10 reps, dead lifting 400 pounds, bench press over 350 pounds.

As a complement to my training, I supplemented pre-workouts with 300 mg of caffeine with a bunch of artificial dyes, coloring and toxins. I took over 10 different supplements for strength gains and low-quality whey proteins with a whole bunch of garbage in it. I WAS CONSUMING OVER 220 grams of protein daily which has been shown to dramatically age you at an exponential rate. Short story is, I was beating my body silly. Just check out the pictures and you decide if I was a beefcake.

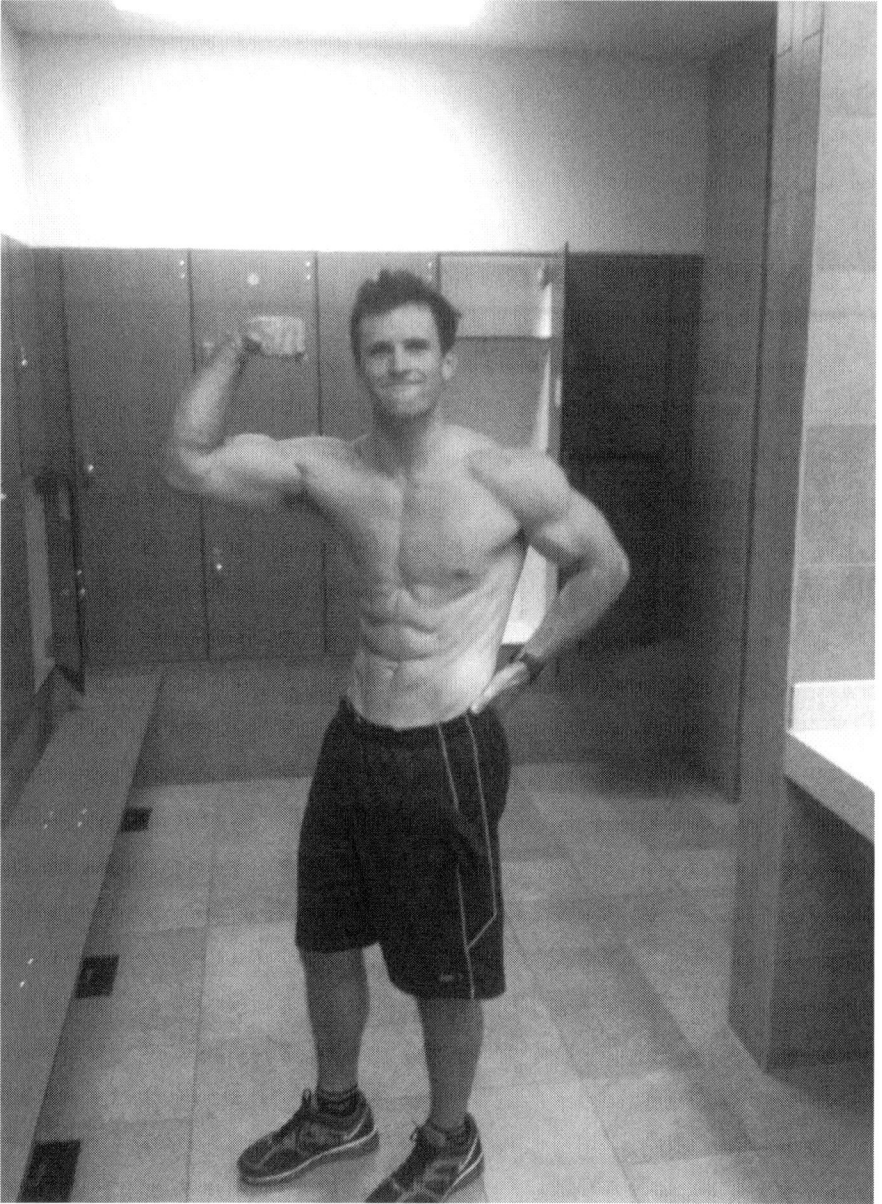

180 pounds, 6% body fat, 2013

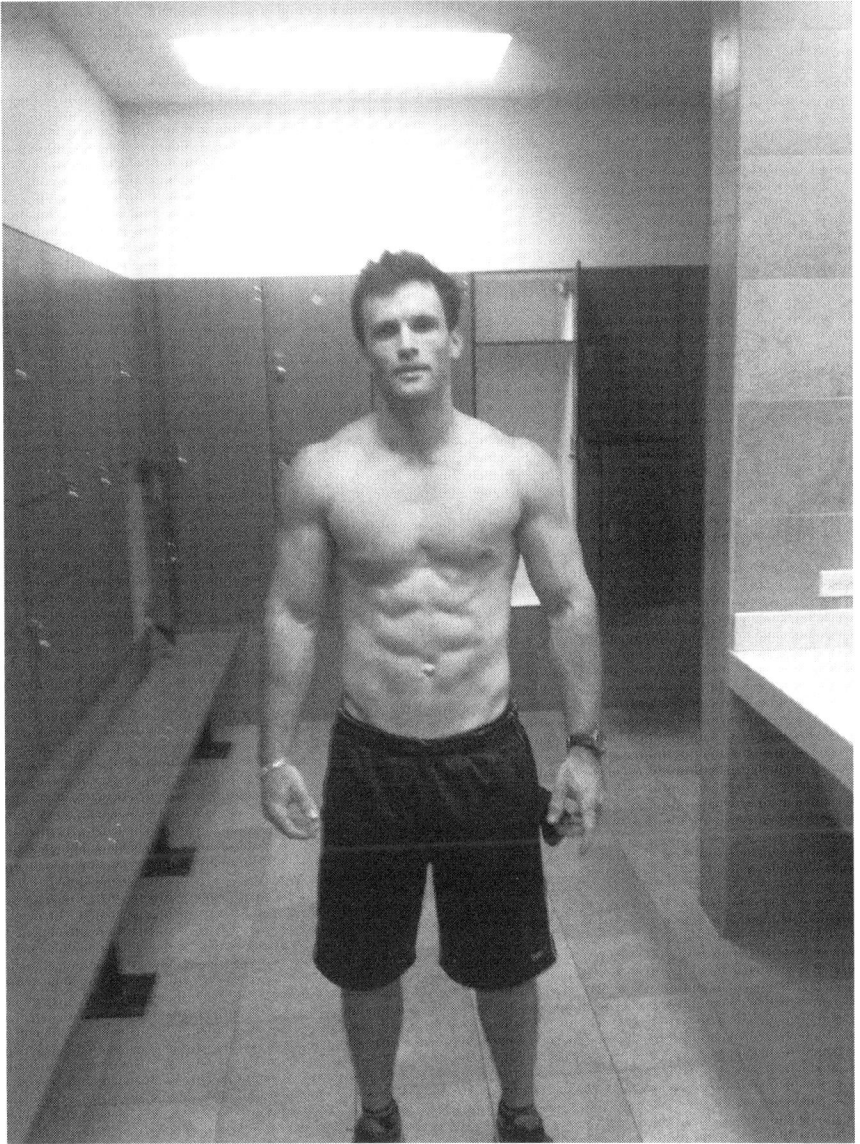

180 pounds, 6% body fat, 2013

Fast forward to April 2014. This is when I embarked on my new journey and was now enrolled at Life University Chiropractic College. However, six months into the program I still carried over some of my bad habits. I was still taking dirty supplements, working out like a fiend and consuming entirely way too much protein.

This continued until at least a year into Chiropractic College. When I finally became fed up with gas, bloating and eczema I decided to try a "detox cleanse" full of bentonite clay, natural laxatives, herbal remedies and a plethora of who-ha-mumbo-jumbo garbage. After two weeks of trying this so-called miracle program I HAD EXPERIENCED THE WORST CASE OF ECZEMA EVER. I was also SEVERELY constipated and had not performed a bowel movement in 4 days. I was in a world of hurt. I had no choice but to seek guidance. I went from 180 pounds with 6% body fat to 140 pounds soaking wet. I was extremely sick.

For as intelligent as people say I am, I was at the time, one of the dumbest humans for not realizing I was ALREADY attending one of the most VITALISTIC and natural healing institutions in the world. This is where I met my mentors Dr. Paul Goldberg and Dr. David Tener who changed my life beyond words. It is through the guidance and lifestyle approaches that are SO EASY to follow that allowed me to clear my skin of Eczema for good.

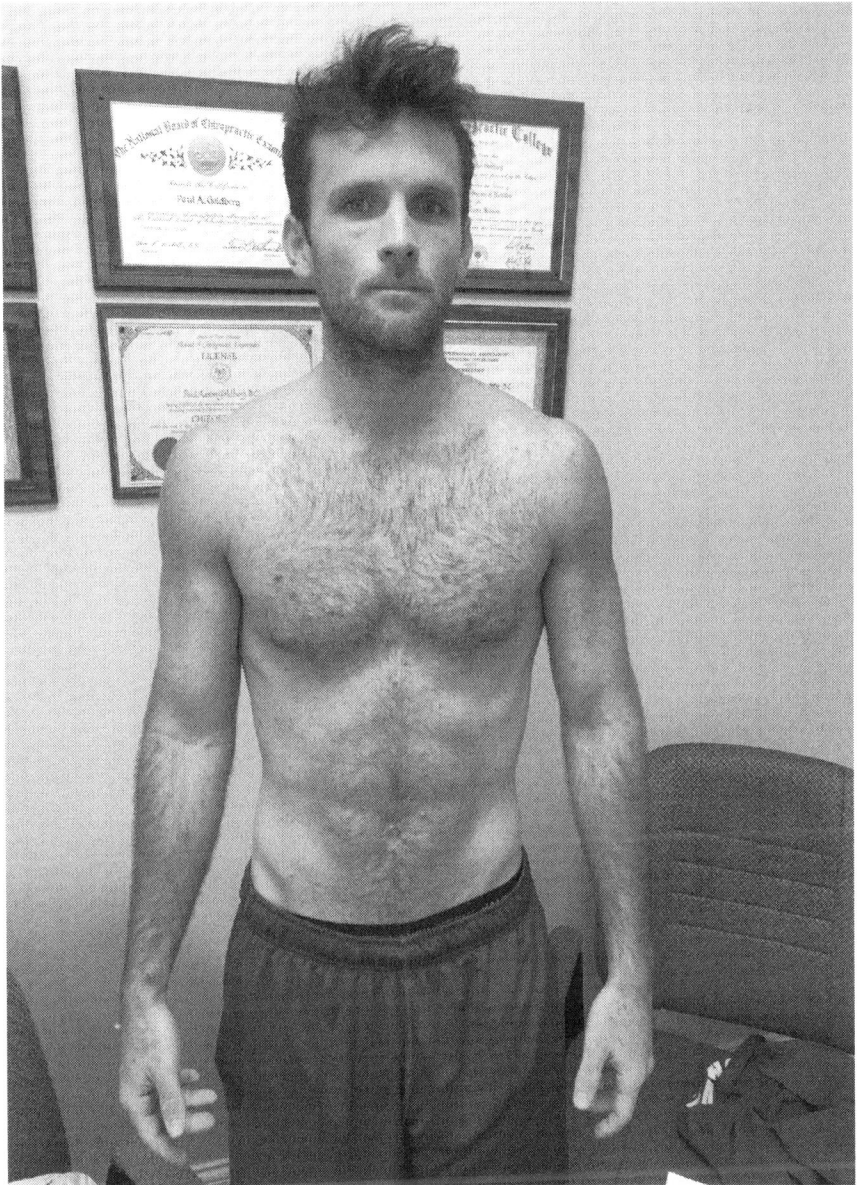

Not seen well in this picture, my forehead underneath my hair was covered with a large patch of oozing eczema. Both arms covered under the hair and my entire chest covered in oozing Eczema. This was the skinniest and lightest I had been since the 4th grade.

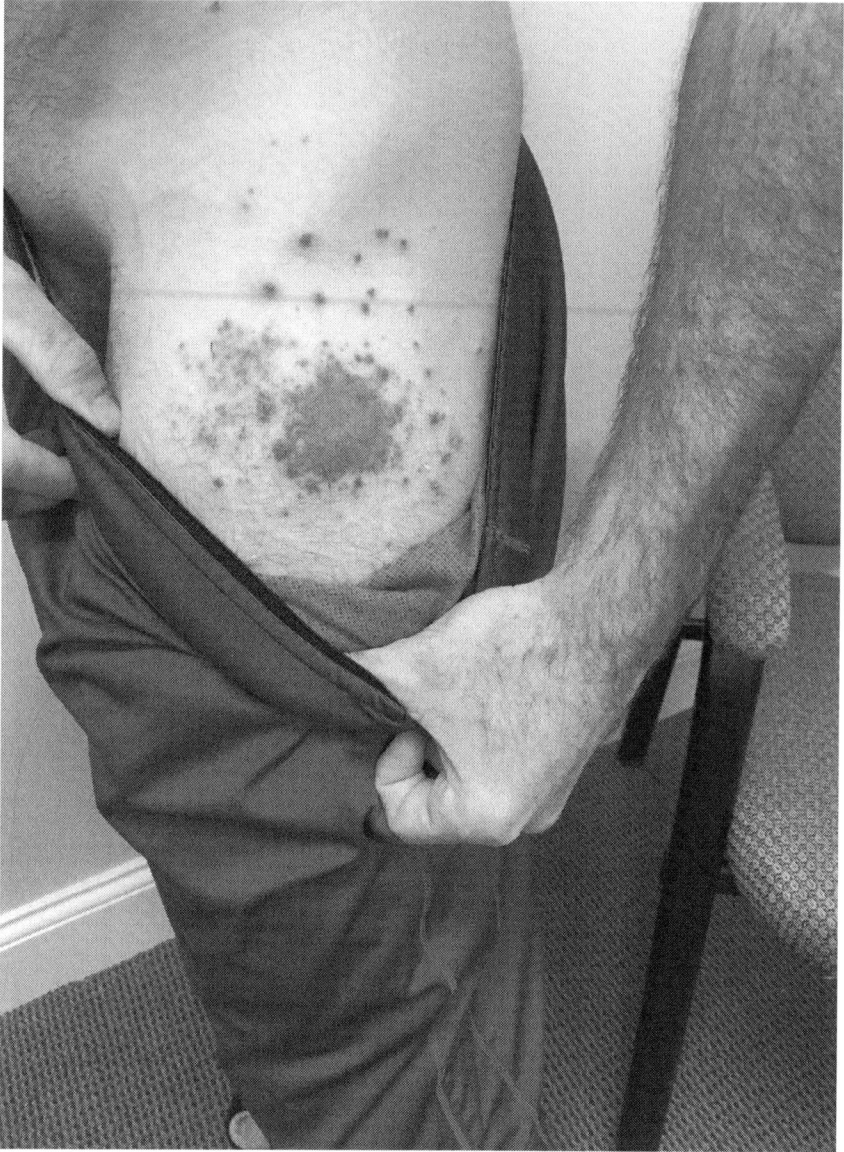

This is a picture of my left thigh completely spread with Oozing Eczema that was relentless. Not shown in this picture was my other thigh and buttocks both covered in Eczema as well. The HARDEST part of my body to eliminate eczema due to lack of air for healing.

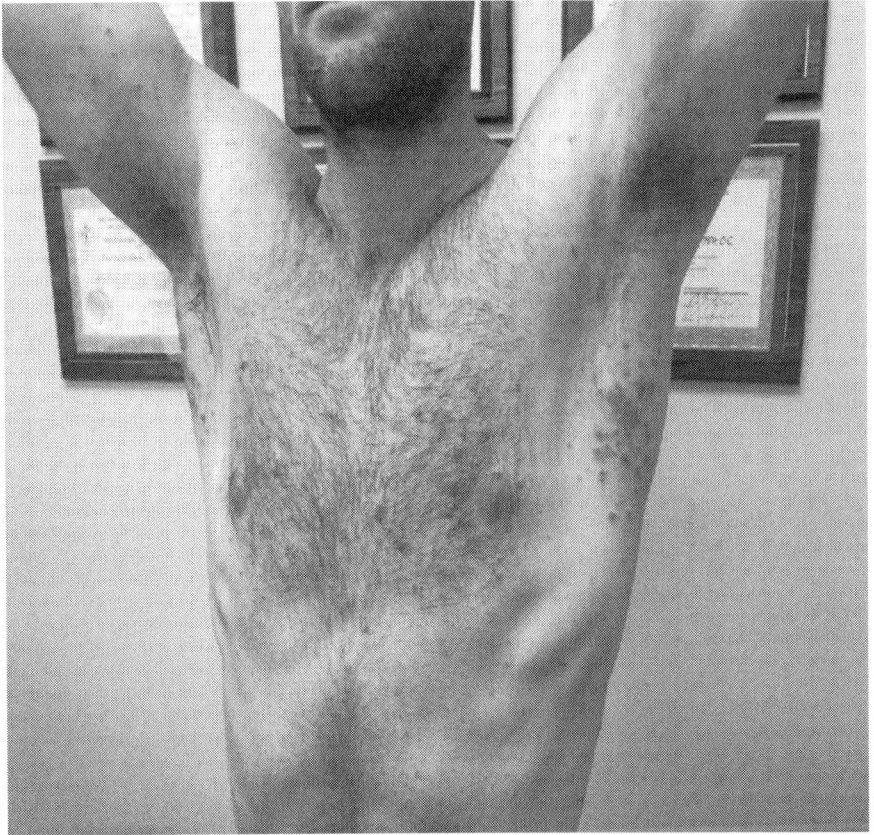

Large patches of Eczema under both armpits and all across my chest. My armpits were constantly stinging due to the pus and sweat. I was severely embarrassed in class when I had to do clinical orthopedic tests and my classmates stared at me as if I was a mutant.

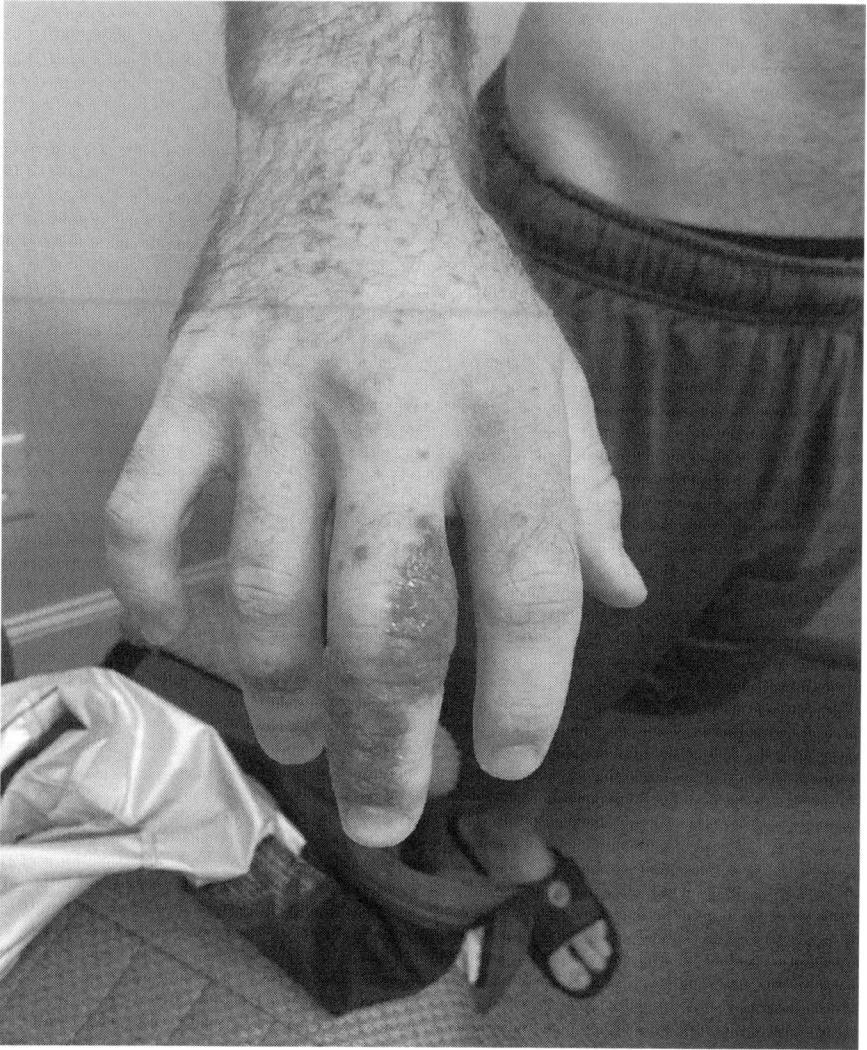

Middle finger and ring finger exploding with oozing and very painful, stinging Eczema that was uncontrollable by any creams or bandages. This was unrelenting and I could feel my finger pulsating when I was under stress.

Through incredible one on one individualistic clinical nutrition, I learned that my small intestine had an overgrowth of bacteria that had been displaced from the large intestine. These bacteria were feeding off digested carbohydrates (sugars) and were creating gas as a byproduct. This lead to systemic inflammation and mal-absorption of vital nutrients and minerals.

Dr. Tenner and Dr. Goldberg flipped my life upside down and taught me all of the things that make us human. The habits I learned are things that we take for granted and now brush off as unimportant.

Instead of living as humans are supposed to, we are now conditioned to seek immediate gratification. To get out of pain fast. Kill illness through antibiotics while destroying all of our good bacteria in the process. We spend 90% of our lives indoors, breathing recycled air. We are losing human companionship through isolation. And we are consuming "Franken-food" which not nutritional value (food created in a lab).

The bottom line was this: I was not absorbing my food, I was not getting enough sunlight, I was overloading my digestive tract with harmful supplements, I was working out WAY too much, I had poor mental health and worst of all, I didn't care. Health is cyclical, just like life. You can always turn it around. You make that decision every day.

Because let me tell you something...

You haven't even come close to your FULL potential.

I officially give you permission to UNLEASH your inner beast.

It only took my body 60-90 days to eliminate my Eczema. And only took a few days to start seeing my skin clear up rapidly. Considering that doctors said, "This is one of worst cases of Eczema they had ever seen", I would say that I had A VERY FAST recovery time. The pictures revealing my Eczema don't even do justice to the amount of pain I went through. The pictures also don't show how red and inflamed I was due to the black and white. If I was one of the worst cases they had seen, and I got these kind of LASTING results, imagine what it will do for you!

Like I said, you can expect to see your skin clearing up WAY before 60 days. But a full clearing of your skin may take up to 60 days. Everyone is designed differently and heals differently. But if you trust the process by sticking to the basics and give it all you have, YOU WILL KILL YOUR ECZEMA for good. Check out the following pictures after only 60 days!

ONLY 60 Days After Implementing Health Goals Designed JUST FOR ME, my chest, my arms, my neck were all completely CLEAR! I no longer had to hide my forehead with my hair because my oozing Eczema was finally gone.

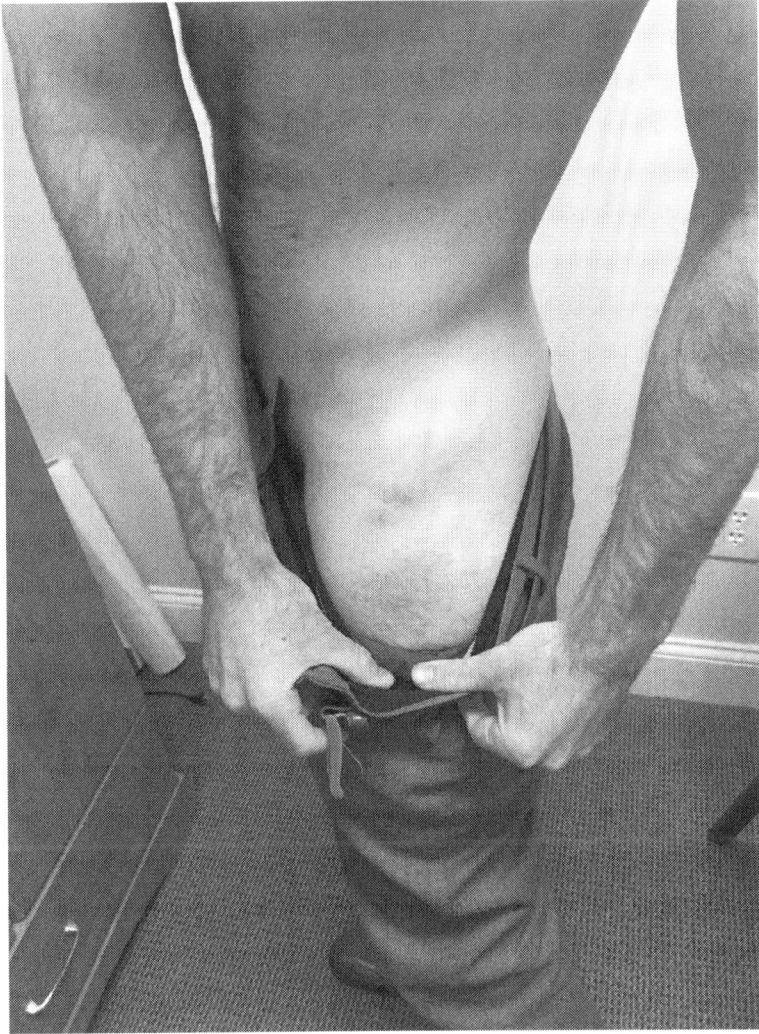

ONLY 60 days after implementing health goals designed JUST FOR ME, I no longer tossed and turned at night as the constant oozing and pain of pus stained my sheets and clothes.

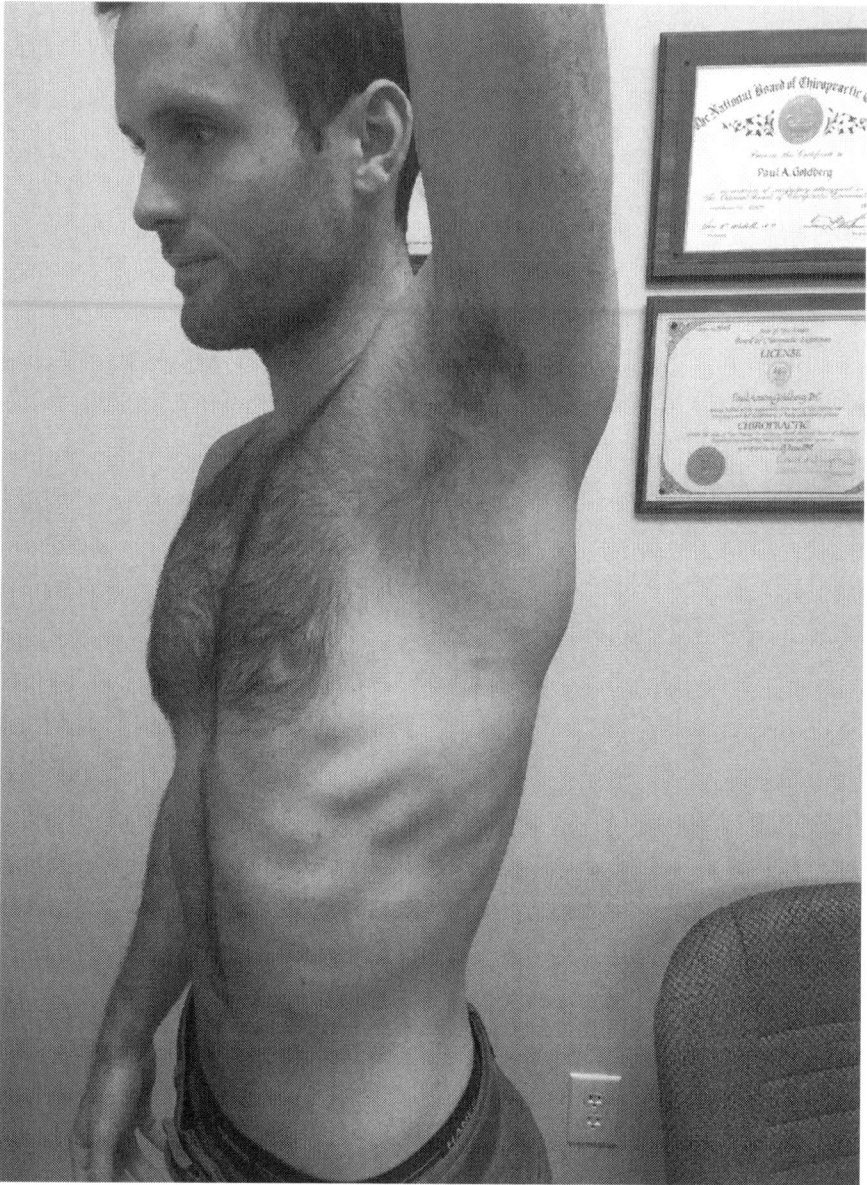

ONLY 60 days after Implementing health goals, I didn't constantly feel the stinging of the oozing opus and sweat running down the sides of my armpits

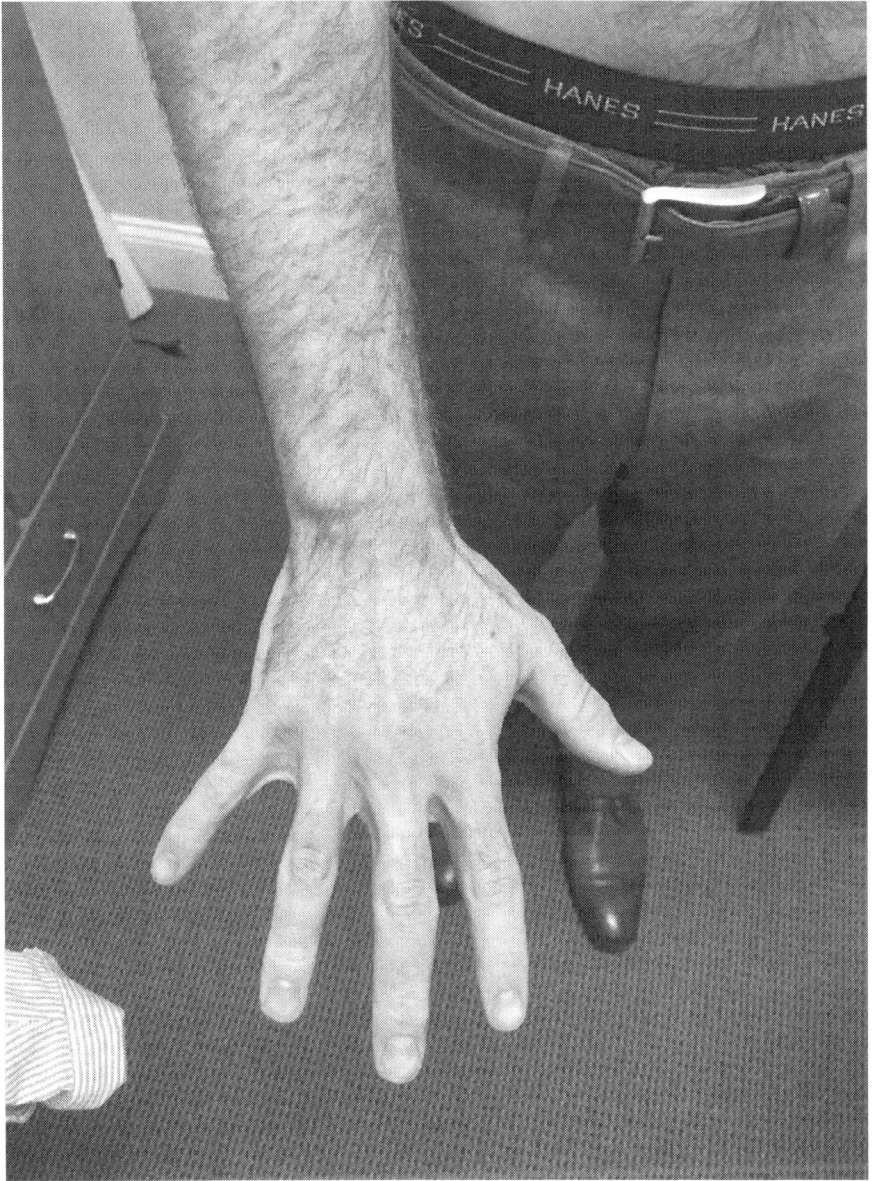

ONLY 60 Days after implementing health goals I didn't have to hide from my classmates during school and avoid the embarrassment of disgust and ridicule. My finger was now usable and didn't sting and throb every time I tried to use it.

My Goals For You:

Understand your mind defines your personal existence.
Create unlimited health potential by the quality of your sleep.
Eat food from the soil.
Realize sunlight is powerful.
Know that relationships matter.
Learn physical appearance does not equate to health.
Find the untapped power you hold and harness it for greatness.

YOUR ROUTINE DEFINES YOU

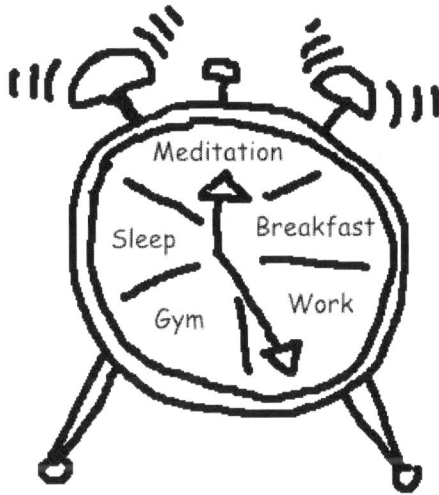

"When you arise in the morning, think of what a precious privilege it is to be alive - to breathe, to think, to enjoy, to love."
- Marcus Aurelius

"WIN THE DAY." This is what my alarm clock has as its caption. Without even knowing it, setting your clock with phrases like "win the day" will allow you to set your day up for success and positivity. It is fascinating how even small words like "WIN" have big impacts on human emotion and psychology. The more we consciously bring ourselves back to positive reinforcement whether through wordplay or positive thinking, we can crush all self-limiting beliefs before they cross the threshold. This will limit the amount of stress we place on our body.

FIRST AND FOREMOST - Before you leave your bedroom I highly recommend making your bed up. I have been doing this since I was 12 years old. It may seem silly, but an activity as simple as this already sets your day up for success. By making up your bed, you have already accomplished something for the day. It is the little tasks that make an even greater impact later. Have you also ever noticed that making up your bed makes your room look and feel 80% cleaner? That's because beds typically take up the bulk of a room and our eyes immediately go to either a messy or a tidy bed. Have you ever also noticed it feels better to be in a room with a made-up bed? That is because psychologically we are able to focus much more efficiently with a room that is kept clean and without the extra clutter. It limits the number of things that our feeble brain has to process. Which, in the digital age, is a lot.

After tidying up your bed, make sure to open your windows and curtains to let the sunshine and outside world welcome you to a new day. Take this opportunity to walk outside for a couple minutes to take a deep breath of fresh air and greet the morning, the sun and surrounding wildlife. Take a moment to gather your thoughts and think how great this day will be, rain or shine. After taking a moment to take in what the morning is offering you, it is time to start your journaling.

Journaling

This is a tactic that I learned from Tim Ferris, although many people before him have utilized journaling as well. No, this is not supposed to be the stereotypical diary. It is more of an objective based manual where you get to track your current thought processes and self-development. It is an excellent place to throw your mind garbage down onto paper and out of your head trap.

Always have a date and time stamped to the top of the entry, this way you can catalogue your journey. I would like to note that you must actually engage in the activity of writing onto physical paper with a pen or pencil and not a computer. By using your hand to write onto physical paper, you are more likely to carry out specific goals and remember your true desires. You are targeting many more brain cell connections when you do this.

Journaling in action:

1st – Begin by mind vomiting onto the paper ANYTHING that comes to mind. Get it all out. It can be how you feel this morning, good or bad. How did the outside make you feel this morning? What did you dream about and how did that affect your morning so far?

Example: *This morning I walked outside to see the sun just peeking above the tree line of my backyard. Wow, was that a sight to see. I already know today is going to be incredible because of how much beauty this day has already given me. I remember last night having a dream that I was standing on top of a mountain looking over the ever-expansive landscape of Earth as I watched the sunset over the Rocky Mountains. The dimming sun light flickered, bounced and danced off of the slow melting caps of ice enwrapped on the rugged peaks of rock. The entrancing rays of light piercing through the low hovering clouds created an exquisite deep pink and orange ambience. It was one of the most tantalizing and simply mesmerizing off-world experience I've had within a dream state.*

2nd - What does your day look like and how do you plan on attacking it? Are there any potential obstacles that may hinder your successful day? What were the things you didn't do so well yesterday that you plan on making better today?

Example: My day looks very busy with many emails to respond to. I plan on responding to only five emails within an hour time frame. The only thing that will keep me from this plan is if I get sidetracked or if I have to meet with a spontaneous client. If this happens, I will just add the remaining emails I didn't get done in that hour and disperse the allotment of emails to each hour thereafter. No biggie!

By first admitting that your day looks busy, then you already consciously know what to expect and you aren't walking into a firing range without goggles and ear protection. You also write down what you anticipate could happen at work so that you won't get flustered if the obvious occurs.

3rd – What are your current goals and desires? How far have you come since first implementing them? What is the current status of those goals and desires? Is there anything that can make those goals come quicker or be of better quality when you achieve them? Refrain from making such overreaching goals at first and celebrate the smaller victories that will lead to the big goal.

Example: My current goal is to get rid of 50% of my eczema by the first month. I am currently two weeks into my goal and my eczema looks better but not exactly where I hoped it would be. Maybe because it was from slipping a little bit on my diet, or I didn't get the sleep that I needed the other night or it was from the stress that I let get to me. Now that I know it was from the stress, I will step away from the activity or engagement that created that stress. Then I will gather my thoughts and realize I am creating thoughts and images in my head that don't exist.

Make sure to also journal before heading to sleep. Log all the things you did great today and the things you didn't do so great. Write down how you can improve on the things you didn't do too well on and how it will affect your happiness and progress of eliminating eczema.

Priming/Meditation

The art of priming and meditation is nothing new in the world of human performance. It can be placed into categories of mindfulness and mindset. The premise is to establish a state of peak performance by tapping into a clear and focused mind to begin the day strong. It is designed to get your body moving in singularity and excitement. If you don't have excitement before your day starts, then how do you expect to be excited at any other time in the day? It is when you practice these drills in the morning that they become part of your routine. You acquire the ability to give birth to a powerful mind, which grants access to a powerful body.

One of the greatest life coaches, spiritual leaders, philanthropists and human beings on this planet is Tony Robbins. During his time on Earth, he has never lost one human to suicide that he himself offered guidance to. He does this by guiding people through their own powerful identity. It's not so much what Tony teaches that makes people reach an enlightenment, it's how Tony gets people to FEEL about their inner power. Tony offers the ability for people to tap into their human physiology to create massive paradigm shifts in their life, health and relationships. The way you perceive yourself, is the way you will perceive the world and everyone around you.

PRIMING IN ACTION:
There are many forms of priming/meditation that you can utilize and they all work very well. The form of priming that I will be showing you is the one that Tony Robbins teaches, as I find it effective.

1. Find a chair to sit in. Find a quite isolated area where you can be away from everyone for ten minutes. Sit up straight without the use of the back support. Feet on the floor, chest up, neck upright, chin parallel with the ground

2. Introduction of breathing patterns – You will be doing 3 sets of 30 rapid breaths. Make sure to get your arms involved in this activity too. Arms above your head as you inhale through your nose and then arms down as you exhale out your nose rapidly. After 30 rapid breaths take 1-minute to rest between the next set. During this 1-minute rest become aware of how your body feels, you may feel a little light headed, tingling in the fingers or feet, this is normal. Then begin set 2 of 30 breaths, then take 1-minute break. Then begin set 3 of 30 breaths, then take 1-minute break.

3. Feel heart beat – place both hands on your heart as you come down from the breathing drill. Feel your heart pump and push all the new oxygenated blood out to all of your vital organs and cells. Hold hands on heart for 30 seconds.

4. Be grateful – After 30 seconds while your eyes are closed, think of 3 things you are most grateful for in your life. It can be a person, past event, something you own, relationships you have, your successes, fortune. It can be as simple as laughing with your family and seeing each of your children's smiling faces. Really focus on these images and step into that image as if you were really there. Then move onto the next thing you are grateful for.

5. Imagine your greatest desire – Visualize the thing you desire most in life. The thing that would give you the most happiness in the world if you were to achieve it. For example: To be completely eczema free, with clear skin and true health. What would that look like and how great of a feeling would that be? Do this for 2 minutes with eyes closed

6. Share the feeling – Share all of the positive thoughts and energy you have culminated over the past few minutes and think about your loved ones and friends. Imagine your

7. friends and family in need of a pick-me up. You then provide them with all of the love and gratitude in the world and they are full of energy and excitement now after you re-invigorated them.
8. Celebrate the desire – Imagine yourself on top of a mountain with a flag in your hand looking over the landscapes of Earth knowing that you accomplished your number one desire: CRUSHING Eczema. Imagine finally defeating the number one thing keeping you back from being fulfilled. You own it!
9. Go take on the day – Take a deep breath in through your nose and out through your mouth. With all of your positive thoughts open your eyes and GO WIN YOUR DAY!!

If you have trouble visualizing or understanding how to do the breathing drills from my above instructions, you can go to YouTube or Tony Robbin's website to watch videos of him performing priming. Just type in "Tony Robbin's Priming Drill or Breathing Exercise."

The time I was left dumbfounded

One of the most prolific concepts I've heard about mindset has altered the way I think about how to live life in the moment. The concept goes like this: "Even when it is cloudy, rainy or stormy outside, the sun is still shining, it's just temporarily behind all of those clouds." This quote is still profound to me. It made me think of what we know about human perception in terms of development.

As children, until a certain age, we lack object permanence. This means that when we are children we only perceive things to exist if they are within our view. For example, from a child's perspective, "If my mother covered her face with her hands, I would think she disappeared and as she uncovers hands from her face, I then see my mommy's face again! Where she went, I have no idea! But I'm so happy she is back!"

Although we gain object permanence as we age, I think we still lack the ability to perceive all that is around us even when we cannot physically see it. We live in a world driven by tunnel vision and forget to experience life in its entirety. We now only focus on what we can immediately see, feel and hear. We zone our energy on what is tangible, certain and apparent. Most of our energy is spent inside of our head, when none of it has sustenance to give us benefit.

The point I am trying to drive home is that the thoughts we make up in our mind are just as powerful as REALITY. Our thoughts, desires and ideas can swallow us alive. We give way too much fuel to generate these false thoughts. The truth is, human action is the only true expression of an idea. All the other clutter in your head is MEANINGLESS! Ideas and thoughts can never be made physical until a person physically carries them into human action. Stop feeding your mind negativity. You will never thrive without first having a healthy headspace.

In the example of a cloudy day – Realize the sun isn't gone, the world isn't ending. Pain and suffering is only temporary. It is your choice to determine how you interpret a rainy day. There is always a rainbow at the end of a rain cloud. Don't get caught up in the darkness of clouds. Sunlight will always penetrate deeper than the largest rain drops.

Routines Summary:
1. Create a motivational caption for your alarm clock to get you juiced up for the day!
2. Open your blinds, windows and curtains to let the sunlight pour into your room in order to welcome the day.
3. Make up your bed before leaving your room. It gives you an automatic sense of gratification and accomplishment. You already have one task for the day!

4. Walk outside to breathe in the fresh air and great the morning. Take a moment to think how excellent the day will be.
5. Begin journaling anything that is on your mind. Whether it is from a dream you had or how you feel this morning. Write down how your day looks and what obstacles could happen that you will overcome. Write down what your current goals are and what the status is of those goals. How can you make those goals come faster? Refer to the section above if you need greater insight or examples.
6. Priming. Prime your physiology. Allow yourself to become tuned into how your body feels by Tony Robbin's breathing and mindset drills. Refer to steps 1-8 mentioned earlier.
7. Your mind can be your worst enemy or your greatest ally. It is a place that is filled with powerful imagery. Remember you control your thoughts. They only exist when you give meaning and action to them. Don't feed negativity, hone it to your advantage.

SLEEP: MORE THAN JUST A DREAMWORLD

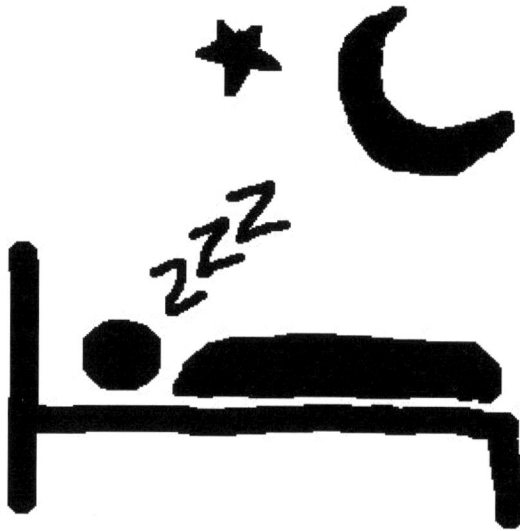

"Sleep is the best meditation."
- Dalai Lama

In a perfect world where we could come and go leisurely without having jobs to attend to, we would wake up with the cycles of the sun and moon. However, our evolved environments have displaced humans into unnatural wake and sleep cycles. We must now set alarms to get us up instead of the noise of the surrounding wildlife or the piercing of the morning sunlight creeping into our rooms.

The way humans now live their lives, sleep has become an option and not so much a requirement. We claim to have what people are calling "Chrono types." Chrono types are explained to be the propensity for a human to sleep and wake up at individual times during a 24-hour circadian clock. In other words, you are either a night owl or a morning person. Once again, human nature claims to know more than what nature and the universe founded us on.

Quite simply put: Humans were designed to wake up when the sun glimpses the surface of your skin's photoreceptors and go to sleep when darkness falls upon Earth. This idea of having more productivity late into the nights or not being able to function in early morning is simply human nature's proclivity to making excuses.

The true nature behind being a night owl or a morning person is from our own perpetuance of pushing our bodies into cycles that aren't innately born into us. We are quite literally mutating our genes. It is something we call evolution. But not a good evolution. Typically, evolution works to help a group of individuals. This, from either using a human attribute more often or not using something as often. Overtime, one human attribute (like our use of an opposable thumb) may get much stronger, while another attribute like our appendix may eventually become obsolete in human anatomy.

However, have you stopped to take notice how sick and nearly dead the human population is? Even during a time where we have the most advanced medicine and technology to date. Our use of evolutionary decisions seems to be shaping us into a direction of SICKNESS and ever spiraling away from WELLNESS.

Sleep, next to food and water, is the most nutritious thing we can provide for our body. Sleep is the only reason we can store memories. It is the only way we can return hormone cycles back to normal after stressful days. It is the only way our body rebuilds itself from the foods we eat. There is a reason why you were always told to read a book before bedtime. It is because you are much more likely to store the information you learn before bedtime than you would if you didn't follow reading with sleep. Your brain must rest for it to process everything you acquire within the day.

Researchers are now saying that a quick 10-minute nap is incredibly beneficial for productivity and memory recall. This, mainly due to all of the many distractions we have in our world today, which is sending our brain into overload. Our brains need rest so that we can bounce back from repetitive strenuous mental processing. Although we are pushing our brains to the limit at times, our brain doesn't get enough credit these days. The common misconception that we only use 10% of our brain is silly. We certainly do use the entire brain. However, each part of the brain is allocated to certain or more specialized tasks at certain times.

For instance, the cerebellum forms the base of the brain which is responsible for your balance and coordination, while the frontal lobe of your brain is responsible for problem solving and actually figuring out your desired body movement. As I'm writing this now, I'm using more of my frontal lobe in order to figure out my next sentence on the paper, while my cerebellum is keeping me upright in my chair without me consciously thinking about it. Make sense?

Now back to sleep – As I've stated earlier we live in a tech savvy world. People now check their Facebook about 50 times a day, Instagram 100 times, Twitter 80 times and their cell phones easily 500 times daily. I'm also taking into account that my numbers are actually underwhelmingly low. These numbers are probably on the low scale of tech addiction. Regardless, the point is that we are in a world run by artificial intelligence and the light that is emitted from these devices doesn't bode all too well with human physiology and sleep.

In the realm of sleep, blue light wavelength, which is the light that comes out from your cell phone, computer, tablet, TVs and ceiling light bulbs affect your sleep cycles. Technically after the sun goes down in the evening, we should be preparing for bed within the hour. Yes, this means that if the sun sets at 5:30pm you should be in bed by about 7pm. Now, this is what "normal" circadian rhythms suggest for humans and I do not expect or ask of you to be in bed at that time. But we are no longer abiding by our true clocks and we stay up way past the sun goes down.

The blue light that comes out from our devices are artificially emulating sunlight. This means that subconsciously when we blast that light into our eyes before we go to sleep at night, our bodies perceive it as being daytime still and WILL affect your sleep. This can either make it harder to go to sleep or stay asleep. When blue light touches your skin or enters your eyes it automatically stimulates the cortisol pathway in our body. This is why we wake up when sunlight enters our rooms in the morning.

Cortisol is our naturally circulating stress hormone. When this hormone is continually pumped through the blood stream it keeps us awake, creates more stress to the bodily organ systems and can lead to chronic disease overtime. Having an overabundance of cortisol in the blood will shut off the production of the natural hormone melatonin. Melatonin is responsible for the quality of our sleep. It allows us to enjoy deep sleep and relaxation. That being said, cortisol and melatonin are in direct competition for your attention and sleep.

I understand there is much to get done for some people before heading off to bed and there is no way around that. I do, however, have a bio-hack that many people utilize to get the most out of their night without sabotaging their circadian rhythms. There are glasses you can purchase for next to nothing that blocks the artificial blue light. They are typically called "blue-light blocking" glasses. There are many companies selling stylish forms if that suits your fancy. I personally only use them for at home use about an hour before I head off to sleep to start the melatonin cycle. Others wear them out at night if they are going to a social event. The choice is totally yours. However, I do believe you will see a big jump in your sleep quality by trying them out during the night and before bed. You can find them on Amazon.

I will also recommend to darken your room as much as you can by purchasing black out curtains. This is to make sure you are not awoken or disturbed by light. Studies have shown that if light touches your skin it will create a physiological response and can wake you up. This is because we also have photoreceptors on our skin.

You also want to sleep in a cool climate. Typically, 65-70 degrees Fahrenheit is favorable for sleep. At these temperatures, many studies point to greater sleep and excellent hormone cycling. Studies have shown a significant increase in testosterone in men while sleeping in cooler climates. If you get cold, just throw on more blankets!

Regardless of daylight savings time, I generally recommend being in bed by 9pm and asleep by 10pm. For some of you that may seem absurd! That's totally okay. If you typically go to bed at 12pm then try for 11pm first and then work your way down to 10pm. I don't expect you to jump in all at once. I do expect you to eventually adopt the lifestyle. You will see massive changes in your mood, relationships, energy and outlook on life. You will no longer dread the alarm clock in the morning because you will most likely wake up before the alarm goes off, I know I do.

When we get to the section on nutrition I will tell you to make sure to eat your dinner or any food 3 hours before going to sleep! You will thank me later.

Sleep Recap:
1. When you have trained yourself, be in bed by 9pm and asleep by 10pm. If you stay up until 12am usually, then try going to sleep at 11:30pm the next night. Then 11:00pm and then 10:30pm and so on. You will get used to it as your progress along.
2. Refrain from the overuse of digital devices such as your cell phone, computer, tablets and TV as these will synthetically stimulate cortisol release, making it hard to fall and stay asleep.
3. If you are going to look at your devices at night, I highly recommend purchasing blue-light-blocking glasses off Amazon. I personally use the $10 UVEX glasses that look like construction worker eye protection. Put on these glasses when it gets dark outside and then take them off when you plan to go to sleep.
4. Back out your room for zero light to enter.
5. Turn your thermostat down to 65-70 degrees Fahrenheit at night.
6. Eat your last meal three hours before going to sleep for high quality sleep (covered later). If you plan to close your eyes at 10pm, finish your last bite by 7pm.

Nutrition: Eat the Earth

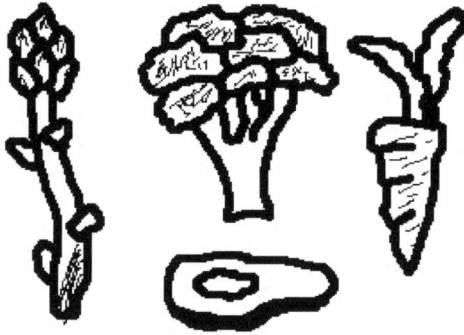

"Our bodies are our gardens – our wills are our gardeners."
-William Shakespeare

"True healthcare reform starts in your kitchen, not in Washington"
-Anonymous

I will preface this section by saying that I get passionate regarding nutrition and in the way that our world currently deals with sick care. I mean no disrespect in any way, shape or form if you feel offended at any given point. The dietary approach that I share with you is indeed the exact approach I took to get rid of my eczema for good. The opinions I express in the upcoming reading comes from how one of the greatest countries on planet Earth continues to feed its people false information. The leaders of health care in America continue to cater to big pharmacy and big agriculture. It's strictly profit. There is no game to be played without having sick Americans first.

The land of pills, potions, medicine, diet fads, weight-loss tricks, anti-aging and health gurus. How many more times are you going to be led astray? How many more times will you be tricked? How much more money will you shower onto the medical community. How many more super-food, detox concoctions will you try until you realize health isn't something that is obtained overnight.

We have been trained to seek immediate pain relief from pain killers, antibiotics, antacids, laxatives, surgeries, autoimmune TNF blockers and topical steroid creams. When DID WE EVER NEED this when we lived in the wild? The answer is NEVER. Does no one ever think to get to the root cause of their condition? The answer, again, is no. Why would you figure out the root cause when you can take a pill to mask everything and forget about it? Seems like a perfectly logical approach as your health spirals into the toilet, am I right?

The approach is straightforward:

STOP consuming foods that have no nutritional value and stop eating so much. When did we think it was a good idea to make and consume food that is entirely made of synthetic sugar and cover it in chocolate? Oh, and then put some caramel and peanut butter inside it. When did we decide to create a carbonated drink made of water(barely) and 65 GRAMS OF SUGAR in one bottle?! When did we decide that you must have breakfast, lunch and dinner in one day? When we lived in the wild we were lucky to eat once a day! I think it's when we decided that we wanted to create the biggest health crisis our world has ever seen. Nearly 1/3 of the United States alone is obese and has diabetes. What kind of life is that? Meanwhile, big pharma and big medicine are licking their chops as they see big profits. They prey on sickness! There is no money in wellness care!

Now, my approach to finally getting rid of your eczema is actually very straightforward, as mentioned before. There are no gimmicks or magic potions to consume. Each person was built to be an individual. Each person was born with certain traits both physiologically and anatomically. Which means healing times and approaches for each person WILL VARY! The nutritional guidelines I give you at this stage are only GUIDELINES and tweaks may need to be done.

I will say from experience, best results come from individual lab testing. This means that as a health care provider, I highly recommend you participate in one-on-one coaching with me if you can. This will give me more information through specific lab tests based on your unique presentation. Don't fret! Even if you follow the plan I give you, there will be incredible results. It just may take a tiny bit longer as you have more room for slacking off. Whereas if you were to coach with me, you will have someone to confide in, express your slip-ups and get back on the crazy train to health! I will be your buddy, guide and mentor whenever you need it.

Let me ask you a question. Have you ever participated in a so called "Detox" that claims to have helped thousands of people including your friends? But when you tried it out you got zero results or even made your symptoms worse? The reason why you may have not responded well to a certain "Detox" but one of your buddies did awesome on the "Detox" is because they either got lucky or certain ingredients inside of the "Detox" did not agree with your digestive tract. This is an excellent example of individuality. Not everyone is built the same way. People have different healing times and needs. Lab testing is the gold standard for understanding your uniqueness.

Please let me express my sincerity and I mean no offense when I say, the medical community has zero training in clinical nutrition. This is, of course, unless they have attended a weekend seminar or certification course. They do not learn nutrition within medical school. They learn pharmacology (drug pushing).

Chiropractors, on the other hand, get MANY HOURS of nutrition and learn how to take care of the body with what the Earth already provides in its natural state. Again, I do not intend to put down medical doctors in any way. They are excellent at what they were taught and are phenomenal in their scope of practice. What is exciting, however, is the past couple years most medical doctors are turning to functional medicine which deals with more food and less medical approaches. Many doctors are realizing just how sick our world is becoming from the nasty pharmaceutical stranglehold. It is refreshing to hear they are choosing to lead their patients down a road of true health from the inside out.

BEFORE YOU EVEN CONSIDER STARTING THIS PLAN

IF YOU HAVE ANY PRE-EXISTING AUTOIMMUNE DISEASE OR CONDITION THAT IS SERIOUS ENOUGH TO BE ON MULTIPLE MEDICATIONS PLEASE DO NOT START THIS PLAN WITHOUT

FIRST CONSULTING YOUR CURRENT MEDICAL DOCTOR.

PLEASE BE ADVISED: IF YOU HAVE OR HAD ANY HISTORY OF CANCER, PLEASE CHECK WITH YOUR MEDICAL DOCTOR OR SPECIALIST BEFORE ATTEMPTING ANYTHING I RECOMMEND HERE.

IF YOU ARE SICK OF WHAT YOUR MEDICAL DOCTOR HAS TO SAY AND WANT TO SCHEDULE A ONE-ON-ONE CONSULT WITH ME TO DISCUSS YOUR OPTIONS, BY ALL MEANS, PLEASE REACH OUT TO ME.

AGAIN: PLEASE DO NOT ATTEMPT OR CONTINUE THIS PLAN IF YOU HAVE A SERIOUS MEDICAL CONDITION IN WHICH YOU ARE NOT FIT TO TAKE A RADICAL CHANGE IN YOUR CURRENT STATE.

ONE MORE TIME FOR CLARIFICATION: You MUST contact me if you have any condition for which you are currently taking medications. This includes any condition that may contraindicate or hinder your ability to undergo a diet of any sort! If you are aware of any food that I recommend eating that you are currently allergic to, you **MUST avoid such foods**. If you are currently anemic, currently having spells of dizziness, or any other condition that is being monitored by a medical doctor **YOU MUST CONTACT ME BEFORE PROCEEEDING.**

If you have decided to move forward, I will advise you to stop taking ALL supplements you are currently taking. Only adhere to the supplements I provide for you. The only exception will be if you are currently taking medications or supplements for other conditions that are imperative for your health. We want to eliminate all chance for anything to aggravate your digestive tract by limiting the number of things you are consuming. **AGAIN** – please do not continue if you have a serious medical condition that you are taking medications for. Thank you.

Before I show you this meal plan, please do not feel like you need to jump into it right away. As I stated in the beginning of the book, I don't want you to quit because it is such a radical change in your diet. For instance, if you drink one can of carbonated beverage a day then try to only have one carbonated beverage every other day. Then only one carbonated beverage a week until you no longer are drinking carbonated beverages.

Take baby steps until you are ready to take the challenge head on. **Do the same with coffee and tea**. Now, I do not have problems with coffee and tea but for the purposes of this program we need to eliminate all risk of stomach irritants. Although caffeine has great benefits, it could also be affecting your digestive tract in ways you may not be aware of.

Off We Go

The meal plan will be broken down in steps at the end of the book for greater clarity and accessibility. This next part is a descriptive break down of your meal plan.

FIRST WEEK: Let me first start by saying the first week your "diet" will consist of only a rice protein powder that I SPECIALLY FORMULATED. If you have not purchased it yet, I highly recommend you get it, as it is crucial for your healing. You can contact me directly to purchase it or can get it off my website. The rice powder will be mixed with 8oz of water. You will drink this rice protein 3 times a day. Morning, afternoon and dinner.

IF YOU DID NOT PURCHASE THE UNLEASHED HUMAN RICE PROTEIN: PLEASE REFER TO THE OTHER PLAN OF ATTACK AT THE END OF THE BOOK (CHAPTER: Your Metamorphosis Begins Here: Your Most Ultimate Transformation.)

PLEASE DO NOT THINK THIS IS A DETOX FORMULA. Because it is not. The rice protein will be accompanied by a multivitamin, vitamin C, and any other supplements dependent upon your lab testing. You will also have the option to drink vegetable broth. I have added the recipe and directions for the broth on page 51.

The purpose of the first week is to allow your digestive system to **REST**. It has taken a beating from all of the harsh detoxes and foods that it has been bombarded with over your lifespan. Our goal is to let things settle as this first week begins. It is our way of letting old tissues that line your stomach to detach and be expelled from your body. This will pave the way to allow your digestion to rebuild itself with strong and healthy cells.

THE FIRST WEEK WILL BE CHALLENGING. YOU WILL BE HUNGRY. YOU WILL HAVE DREAMS ABOUT DONUTS AND BAD FOODS. You will feel very guilty in your dreams. But you will wake up feeling relieved that you didn't cheat in real life! It was all a dream! Trust me, it will happen, because I experienced this first hand.

You will be tempted to eat solid food during this time. Resist the urge! Just remember what your goals are. Remember what your desires are. This is when mindset and meditation drills become extremely important. PLEASE, PLEASE, make sure to drink ALOT of water! There will be times that you feel lightheaded from a seated position, to a standing position. This happened to me as well. It is normal, as your body is going through many changes quite quickly. Just take your time in the first week. Limit physical activity. Do not work out in the gym. I recommend you taking light walks around your neighborhood, but nothing more!

IF YOU CAN OR ABLE TO TAKE A WEEK OFF FROM WORK I HIGHLY RECOMMEND DOING IT.

If you can't take off a full week, take of Weds-Friday. This will give you a nice start so that you can have Saturday and Sunday to rest. This will limit the amount of activity and stress you are placing on your body. I'm not going to lie, it will be tough, but you are only suffering short term for long term victory.

Vegetable broth:

Vegetable broths have been utilized since the time of Hippocrates and play a vital role in the replenishment and growth of new tissue. This was a tremendous supplement to the rice protein during my healing process. It provided me an excellent source of vitamins and nutrients extracted from the vegetables. It also gave me another food source to consume, which was a **LIFESAVER.**

Directions:

Bring a quart of purified water in stainless steel pot to a boil. Once water is at a boil:

Add 3 chopped up carrots

Add 2 chopped up zucchinis

Add 2 chopped up yellow squashes

Add Two bunches of parsley

Add green leafy vegetables such as collards or kale

1. Cook at a rolling boil for 15 minutes and then let it simmer for an additional 60 minutes covered.

2. Let it set for a bit before consuming, as it will be hot.
3. Strain out the vegetables and pour the broth into either glass mason jars or glass containers. **DO NOT** eat any of the vegetables, as all the nutrients have been leached from them.
4. Do not add any spices or extra ingredients to the broth.
5. Only a pinch of Himalayan sea salt is permitted.

You can make this broth in bulk and store it in the refrigerator up to four days at a time. If you are to heat up the broth, refrain from using the microwave. Instead, use the stove top. Microwaves are nasty creations. If you have one, stop using it. They distort food particles that are not conducive for any animal on Earth to consume. More on this later. Just know microwaves are not your friend – ever.

SECOND WEEK: Depending on your progress, beginning the second week you will start a diet on a **STRICT non-starchy** vegetable-based diet. Non-starchy means vegetables that don't contain high carbohydrate content. Vegetables with higher carbohydrate content are typically harder to break down and require many more enzymes to break them down into smaller food particles.

We want vegetables like ORGANIC salad greens, carrots, asparagus, radishes, kale, cucumber and brussels sprouts. **Always, always** steam your vegetables. Do not eat them raw. You want to make digestion as easy as possible. Raw vegetables are much harder to break down than cooked vegetables. Never char your vegetables as the burnt ends will create inflammation in your body due to free radical formation/oxidation. I will provide a list of the foods, spices, oils and additives you CAN and CANNOT eat in later chapters. I will also list the foods to ALWAYS avoid. During this phase, you should continue to take your rice protein 3x a today along with your recommended supplements.

Very important for the second week going forward
CHEW YOUR FOOD TO A PULP.

When you are implementing solid food back into your diet, it is crucial for you to eat slow and chew a lot! I know this is going to sound crazy, but make sure to chew your food at least 100 times before swallowing. Now I am going to be honest, in the beginning I actually want you to consciously count the chews. Believe me, it seems like a nuisance to count the number of chews, but over time you will get used to it and it will become a new normal without even counting. You will have been trained so well to chew your food, that you won't even think about it anymore.

This act of chewing was coined by Horace Fletcher, who found that by chewing enough and chewing slow, he was able to heal his own unhealthy habits and ailments. Horace Fletcher at 5 feet 6 inches, weighed two-hundred and seventeen pounds. He was ridden by indigestion, frequent influenza and had white hair at the age of 40. Keeping ALL of his other lifestyle choices constant he decided to just chew slowly and chew well. To his astonishment, by chewing his food very well, he lost sixty pounds of fat. His head was the clearest it had ever been. He had not been sick for the whole year and his constant feeling of lethargy was gone. He tried to spread the word of his success to everyone, but nobody believed his voodoo nonsense. This was until he converted a medical doctor into a believer.

This medical doctor was Dr. Van Someren. Van Someren was a very ill man. He had been sick for nearly 3 weeks. He was skeptical of Horace, but with all other medical approaches exhausted, he decided to take a chance. Horace introduced clean organic foods and instructed Dr. Van Someren to eat slowly with many chews. It wasn't but a few days that Dr. Van Someren was set free of his ailments. It was at this point that they began publishing scientific articles on the subject. These articles were published within the

British Medical Association on the subject of proper mastication of food and the impact of overall health in humans.

When you chew your food enough it releases natural enzymes from your salivary glands and your pancreas. This allows your food to be broken down way before it is swallowed. This way your gut has almost barely any responsibility and will continue to allow your digestion to relax. Thus, giving it more time to grow stronger each day. Also, make sure to NEVER drink liquids during a meal! If you are chewing your food enough and eating slow enough you should never need to drink fluids during a meal. When you drink fluids during a meal it will neutralize the stomach acid and make your body more basic. Our bodies are naturally acidic and when you decrease stomach acidity it decreases the effectiveness of digestion. The purpose of stomach acid is not only to break down food, but also to eliminate any bacteria that may sneak into your digestive tract. Therefore antacids like Prilosec OTC, Pepcid, and Zantac are so dangerous. These are medications that are widely abused for conditions like heart burn, acid reflux, indigestion and GERD. They directly neutralize stomach acidity, leaving your digestive tract open for attack from invaders such as viruses and bacteria.

When antacids are chronically abused, bacteria easily slip by our acid defense and allow colonies of bad bacteria to grow. This can lead to leaky gut and a whole slew of autoimmune conditions. Not to mention, you will be sick more often and will likely catch any sickness that is going around. This includes your workplace, your gym and even your children's school.

The mindset approach is simple. If you eliminate the harmful foods and drinks that are causing your indigestion, you don't need to take antacids. Easy peasy right? Again, it is the mind-paradigm-shift people must have to make small changes in their dietary habit. Education is more important than implementation. You must understand why you are adopting a habit before you understand what the habit is and how you are going to do it.

THIRD WEEK: Will be very similar to the second week. We will continue to eat non-starchy vegetables and continue with the rice protein formula. If you are a part of my coaching group we may be able to throw in certain nuts or nut butters. This comes from your lab testing. I will know the foods you can or cannot tolerate based on food allergy panels. Make sure to continue to take the supplements I recommended and the times I designated for you.

FOURTH WEEK: By the end of the month, if you kept true to the food guide and you didn't cheat, you should start to see your skin clear up significantly. At this point, you may consider adding in fish 3 times a week. It should be baked and not grilled! No other animal meat at this point will be allowed. Please make sure the fish is wild caught. You may either bake Salmon or Mahi. You may also find wild canned salmon in the health food store and mix it in salad greens with sea salt and organic olive oil. Remember to chew a lot and to eat slow! Your body hasn't had exposure to this much protein in a while.

I want to keep reiterating that this month will be challenging in the **SHORT TERM**. You will be hungry. You will get tired of foods quickly! However, this is just a phase! It won't last forever. We must keep things simple. It allows your digestive tract to rest. Again, I will provide a list of foods, oils, spices, liquids allowed and those not allowed.

Three Hours before bed
Make sure to eat your last meal three hours before heading to sleep. By eating way ahead of bedtime, your body is able to break down food way before you lay down. It should also be noted that digestion works best if you are letting food flow with gravity.

This means after a meal it is best to sit up in a seat or chair since food will fall down your digestive tract with ease. Even better – go on a nice 15-20-minute walk after dinner!

I will stress, however, that you must not lay down, as this impedes the digestive process. Have you ever noticed that when you lay down after a meal you tend to get burpy or have indigestion? That is because your gut has to work harder to pull and push down the food for it to be digested. Gases get caught in pockets and have nowhere else to go but out of your mouth. This is why you get burpy and gassy when laying down after a meal.

The other important part of eating before bedtime is the digestion process itself. One of the contributing factors of lethargy and sleeplessness is from eating a large meal right before bed time. When you eat right before bedtime, your stomach now has to focus all of its time and energy to breakdown all of that food. It is spending almost 80% of your body's energy to digest food, when it should be targeted for sleep!

This will cause you to toss and turn. You won't get into deep sleep. You might feel stomach pains or burnings. You can have acid reflux or heartburn.

Even if you don't feel immediate affects from food before bed or if you are now completely used to digestive pains, your sleep will remain of low quality. If you practice this new habit of eating three hours before bed, you will finally feel rested and fresh upon waking. It made a big difference for me! Let me know how it turns out for you!

Probiotics

People today are always talking about how they are taking a new probiotic. They say their last one didn't work, or it seemed to make them worse. The problem with blindly taking a probiotic is that you have no idea which strain of bacteria your body truly needs. Most people have heard of the beneficial bacteria that we harbor in our digestive tract. The question is, do you really know what their purpose is and where they are located?

The beneficial bacteria are primarily located in our large intestine. It Is in the large intestine where the last stages of digestion and absorption occur. This is where B vitamins and vitamin K2 are produced. These two vitamins are CRUCIAL for you to be properly nourished and healthy. It is these two vitamins that allow our colon to absorb calcium, support DNA synthesis and protect nerve cell integrity.

That being said, it is very important to get a stool micro test before you take any probiotics. This lab test will tell you which strains of bacteria you are lacking, which strains you have too much of and if you have any pathogenic strains (bad bacteria). This will let you know which probiotic you need! Sometimes you may just need one strain! The issue is when people purchase probiotics that carry strains that they DO NOT need and can cause other bacteria to multiply. This is why some people may have diarrhea, gas, bloating or constipation after blindly buying a probiotic.

If at any time bacteria flows backward into the small intestine from the large intestine, A LOT OF HARM can occur. This is what happened to me and left me with a condition known at Small Intestine Bacterial Overgrowth (SIBO). The bacteria were feeding off sugars I was eating and they were producing an excess of gas (flatulence). Secondary fermentation of sugar was occurring, thus creating systemic inflammation and causing my skin to erupt with eczema. By performing a hydrogen/methane breath test I was able to see a massive overgrowth of bacteria flourishing in the wrong part of my digestive tract! It was from this test that I had to eliminate all sugars, starchy foods and beans. These foods allow bacteria to flourish because they love to feed off these foods.

Dairy

Dairy is not your friend. Not then, not now, not ever. Let the record show that 90% of the world's population is allergic to dairy. Lactose intolerance and dairy allergy are two DIFFERENT meanings.

Lactose intolerance means you have an immediate reaction to dairy products such as bloating, gas, constipation, stomach ache and diarrhea. Dairy allergy means you are allergic to it based off blood tests, but you may not feel an immediate response in symptoms. Just because you don't feel pain or discomfort DOES NOT mean it isn't harming you.

Let me explain the practical reason why dairy should never have been part of the human diet. For this example, we will be referring to dairy cows. Let me ask you a question... Where does dairy come from? From a mother cow. Who is that milk designed for? ....

........For a baby cow (calf)!

Why do we drink milk from another mammal? We are the only other mammal on Earth that drinks milk from another mammal. Have you ever seen a baby cow drinking milk from a human mother? I think not... that would be weird. But it's not weird when we drink from a mother cow? Cow milk has enzymes and nutrients meant for the calf, not for the human. This is why it is not surprising that we are naturally allergic to dairy in all forms: cheese, milk, butter, creams, etc.

Parents and teens, if you didn't know this already, a good chunk of the reason why your teenage child is suffering from acne, eczema and other skin conditions can be blamed on the overconsumption of dairy products. Actually, not even overconsumption, but consumption alone can cause an outbreak of acne and eczema too! Dairy does a number on young children and adults. Although kids can take a beating and bounce back much more efficiently than adults, they are much more sensitive to foods than adults. Almost 95% of the time, any skin breakout or blemish of any kind can be chalked up to something you are eating. You can take that to the bank!

To add even more insult to injury, the milk we are drinking isn't even in its natural form anymore. We now drink milk with added hormones and thickeners. I'm sure you've heard by now of bovine growth hormone (bGH). Since kids started drinking and eating dairy products, young girls have been maturing much faster. They are reaching menarche at earlier ages, with it lasting way longer until old age. Sounds like a science fiction movie. No, it is real life.

Beans, Legumes, Peanuts, Corn
Stay away from these. They are dirty foods that do not belong in your diet even after your eczema is gone. All of these foods contain things called aflatoxins. Aflatoxins are a type of mold toxin that are considered carcinogens (cancer causing). These are things like peanut butter, peanuts, black beans, chickpeas, hummus, pinto beans, lima beans, green beans, peas, soy beans, corn and even some milk and cheese. Eating these foods can actually affect your liver which is how we detoxify foods. Aflatoxins can also induce new food allergies that you didn't have prior to eating these foods. They can induce autoimmune disease reactions such as psoriasis, ulcerative colitis and Crohn's.

These foods also contain things called "Lectins." Lectins are the protective mechanisms that defend these foods from insects, pests, animals and humans. Lectins are virtually indigestible by humans and flow over into our bloodstream because they have nowhere to go. They are typically found on the outside coating of these foods. The coatings protect them from human digestion so when it is finally released from human bowels, it can return to the soil where it belongs. Lectins will very commonly trigger an immune response in your body by pumping out many antibodies to destroy the lectin. Symptoms can include gas, bloating, sharp and burning stomach pains, nausea and even vomiting.

Lectins are one of the biggest contributors to leaky gut. Normally when food scrapes the gut lining, cells are able to rapidly build and repair the digestive tract. When lectins enter the mix, they blunt the repair process and allow undigested food to enter the blood stream. Uh oh. We then become mineral and vitamin deficient because the nutrients we needed from food were not properly digested and absorbed. The body is on high alert and proceeds to evacuate the bowels and stomach acid through both orifices to expel the intruder. Continuous stress on the digestive lining and immune system will lead to breakouts of eczema, brain fog, lethargy, depression, anxiety, autoimmunity, and organ dysfunction.

Sugars and Fruits

Fruits have been given a magical and almost divine spot in our dietary repertoire. People think that because they have their daily fruit smoothie or morning banana that they are somehow superheroes. People still think that antioxidants are at the secret weapon for disease prevention. While I do believe antioxidants are extremely important, I believe they can be consumed much better and more efficiently. The issue with fruits are that they still contain a lot of sugar per serving. Sugar consumption is at the forefront of disease in our world today and we should limit the amount we are indulging in.

Most people are unaware that the fruits we eat today are much different than their ancestors. Fruit has been genetically modified and cross pollinated over centuries to make them taste better, have less seeds and to be more attractive. For instance, bananas, which I don't understand for the life of me why people eat these still, used to be almost completely made of seeds. They weren't even desirable to eat, as they had almost no meat. Now the banana is completely meat and is loaded with sugar. People think they are healthy by eating a banana since they are getting potassium. What is comical about this is that a banana typically only has 350 mg of potassium. On the other hand, ONE LEAF of Swiss chard contains 1350 mg of potassium. The problem is, no one wants to eat Swiss chard because it isn't the tastiest. Story of the American diet, right? Or should I say SAD – Standard American Diet.

The most dangerous food we are facing in today's age is added sugar. Chances are if you have eczema, you have some sort of gut dysfunction and it typically has a bacterial component like I did. Let me also clarify that a carbohydrate is a sugar and a sugar is a carbohydrate. Now that we have that straight, consuming sugars such as pure sugar, cane sugar, honey, molasses, artificial sweeteners and anything else that makes things sweeter is no good for your gut!

The bacteria in your intestines feeds directly off these sugars. As I stated earlier, these bacteria create secondary byproducts which can create the so called "leaky gut." Leaky gut occurs when the mucus membranes and tissue lining of your digestive tract becomes bombarded by inflammatory chemicals so often, that it allows food particles to leak into your blood stream. This is BAD NEWS! If food is detected in the blood stream, your body turns onto high alert and perceives itself under attack! It treats it as if a virus or bacteria has invaded your blood stream. Your immune system kicks out a lot of antibodies to try to eliminate the false invader. If this continues long term chronic systemic inflammation will lead to decreased immune response, frequent infections, organ dysfunction and hormone dysregulation.

Nutrition Recap:
1. We cannot rely on the powers that be to protect us from ourselves. Take matters into your own hands. Take control of what you consume. Treat your body like a garden that needs careful tending to for growth and flourishment.

2. Eat more of nature, eat less of things made in a lab. Eat more organic and less processed foods.

3. Lab testing is recommended. Lab testing is for individuality. Each person has different reasons for their eczema. Don't shoot blindly in the dark. Know what your gut is harboring. Learn how to balance the chaos in your digestive tract.

4. Remember to chew your food 100 times before swallowing! This allows salivary and pancreatic enzymes to build up in your mouth for pre-digestion to occur. This will break down your food before it even reaches your stomach, making the absorption of nutrients much easier, while also taking stress off your digestive tract. Remember Horace Fletcher's amazing turn-around in health from chewing alone!

5. Again, make sure to eat three hours before heading to sleep for incredible sleep quality.

6. Do not drink fluids during a meal! Let your enzymes and saliva do the work. If you chew enough and slowly, you will never need any fluids to help wash down the food. Try getting away from scarfing food down your gullet.

7. Probiotics – Do not take any probiotic blindly. It can lead to more problems. Make sure to get stool samples to determine which bacterial strain you may be lacking or have too much of. You may be surprised what you find.

8. Dairy – To your dismay, milk products will never be something you can call your friend in health. Almost the entire world has an allergy to dairy. It isn't normal to drink milk from another mammal outside of our species. Those enzymes and nutrients are meant for a baby calf, not a human.

9. Legumes, Beans, Lectins – These nasty mold toxins are the culprits for the scraping of your gut lining. They allow food particles to enter the blood stream. Long term exposure to food inside the blood creates immune system overload. Eventually your sensitive immune system can turn on you and create autoimmune conditions.

10. Sugars and fruits – The amount of sugar that is in our food is sickening. We drink 20 fluid ounces of Coca-Cola comprised of 65 grams of sugar. Even the fruits we praise to be healthy because of antioxidants content, have more sugar than they ever had before due to genetic modification. We eat fruit like candy and think we are being healthy. "I've got a news story for you Walter Cronkite…. We're not!"

The Autoimmune Pandemic

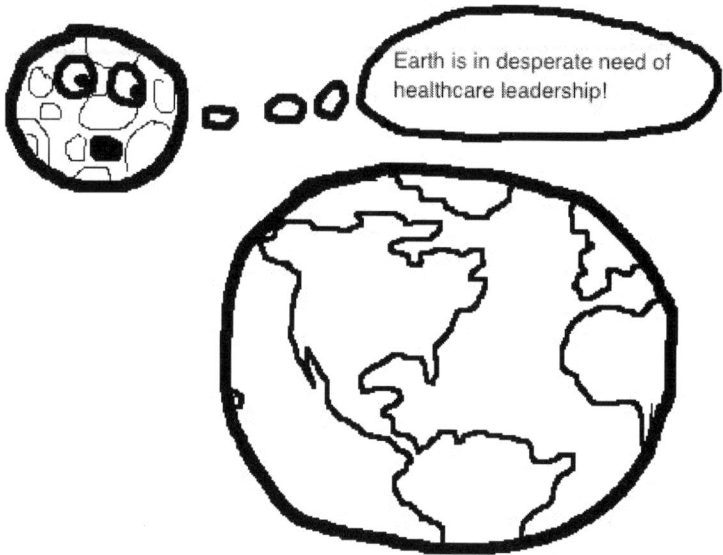

"The Earth does not belong to us: we belong to the Earth."
-Marlee Matlin

We have been trained to react to symptoms as an identifier of health or disease. We believe that if we have zero symptoms that we must be healthy. For example, when we think of a healthy person we imagine someone who is in shape or a fitness model. However, this couldn't be further than the truth. Just like my story when I was cut-up and built at six percent body fat, I was actually super unhealthy.

The body building lifestyle is by no means a model for health. The average gym rat takes very toxic supplements, eats WAY too much protein and stresses their body beyond belief by going to the gym seven times a week. Although some people get away with this lifestyle and have ZERO symptoms now, it is still very much harming their body.

This takes me into my next topic of discussion: Autoimmunity can still be present in your blood and body even if you have zero symptoms.

In the last 30-40 years, autoimmunity (when our body attacks its own healthy cells) has significantly risen. Recent data has shown autoimmunity is rising by nearly 20 percent by roughly every decade. It is important to note that there is a spectrum of autoimmunity. What this means is that autoimmunity is not diagnosed when you start having symptoms, its actually occurring way before you see symptoms.

In the past many years, the U.S. military decided to collect blood samples from millions of service men and women for various reasons. Of importance, there was recently a study of a service woman who had lupus. Lupus is an autoimmune disease that has a cascade of terrible symptoms when it enters deeper phases within the disease. The most well-known symptom of Lupus is typically the butterfly rash on the face.

However, back to the story at hand. This service woman had a blood sample drawn years before she was officially diagnosed with lupus. The lead researcher wanted to evaluate her blood sample from many years before diagnosis. What she came to find from the blood sample was a game changer in the world of autoimmunity.

It is important to note, before I finish this story, that lupus has seven antibodies associated with it, which characterizes the disease when you look at it under the microscope. When all seven antibodies are elevated and noticeable inside the blood, this gives the definite diagnosis for lupus. Well, turns out this service woman had all seven antibodies elevated YEARS before she experienced ANY symptoms AT ALL!

This means that YOUR body could be at risk for ANY kind of autoimmune condition or disease without you even feeling ONE bit of symptomatology! This should be a BIG wake up for you and the world!

Really quick – do you know what the number one sign of a heart attack is? Guess what – IT'S A HEART ATTACK!

So, let me ask you a question. You didn't have pain a week before the heart attack or anything else that would warn you of imminent death, right? So then let me ask you this… Were you healthy a week ago? The answer is NO! The occurrence of a heart attack is the culmination of many years of abuse to your arteries and blood vessels. If you treat your body like garbage, it will treat you just the same. Rant done.

Now, you may be wondering why we have antibodies to our own tissue? When you get a thyroid blood panel, it is usually showing the level of thyroid antibodies and the normal ranges, right? This lets you know your thyroid is either underactive, overactive or normal. It is how we survive.

Antibodies are crucial for us to survive. Our natural antibodies are designed to "take out the garbage," if you will. Our immune system has to get rid of our old and damaged cells to make room for new cells to develop. The way we do that is that our antibodies clear them out. This is when your antibodies are working properly within normal ranges.

On the opposite end, when you have elevated antibodies, this means you are killing off more healthy cells than you are making. This is known as the prodromal phase of autoimmunity (before symptoms begin). This is when your body is being bombarded by antibodies. The body then has the inability to determine which tissue is healthy or unhealthy. So, it decides to delete every single cell and tissue in the body until the host (you) is dead.

AUTOIMMUNITY IS NOTHING TO MESS AROUND WITH. PEOPLE DIE WITH THESE DISEASES. EVERY. SINGLE. DAY.

This prodromal phase goes on for years until you hit the threshold where your body cannot contain it any longer and you start seeing symptoms or in the worst cases, imminent death.

This is the process: You start seeing symptoms and you go to doctor. After you first visit your primary care doctor, it takes two-three years before they even diagnose you with a disease because the symptoms are so minimal that doctors aren't sure which disease you have. At that time, doctors are scratching their heads trying to scramble and figure out what you have, so they give you a broad-based medication to take care of multiple symptoms. You are on these medications for on average three years after symptoms first arrive before you find out you have diseases such as rheumatoid arthritis, ulcerative colitis, Crohn's, Hashimoto's Thyroiditis, Lupus and the list goes on.

What is shocking is that clinically speaking, you will find six to seven out of every ten patients have elevated antibodies to their own tissue if you do the correct lab testing. THIS IS SCARY. Meaning that 60-70% of people today have elevated antibodies in their blood connected to autoimmune diseases WAY before they even see symptoms.

The most dangerous type of antibodies are those called Antinuclear Antibodies (ANA). This is because, as the name describes, they are directly attacking the nucleus of your cells. The nucleus in our cells is the main control center. When this is shut down, a cell dies. The reason I bring this up is because ANAs are very closely linked to all of the environmental toxins that our bodies accumulate in the world we live in now. Toxins like BPA, mercury, radon gas, mold, PCBs, and the list goes on. The problem is that these toxins don't only pass through our respiratory system, they flood our blood stream and start accumulating in our tissues. These toxins will begin to cross react with each other and will magnify the obliteration of health tissues until your immune system reaches its threshold and express very severe health concerns.

The issue currently is that the medical community wants to study each toxin individually. They categorize the typical symptoms associated with mold exposure or inhaling toxic carbon monoxide. The problem is we DON'T live in a world where we are exposed to "just one toxin." This isn't realistic. We currently live in a world where we have multiple toxins that cross react and have an accumulation affect. This creates confusion for doctors today. The doctors think, "someone couldn't possibly be exposed to more than one toxin, my textbook from medical school says they must have this symptom and this reaction." GET YOUR HEAD OUT OF THE BOOKS AND DEAL WITH THE PERSON IN FRONT OF YOU!

One of the coolest things I've heard in a while is from Dr. Thomas O'Bryan who said, "The most common source of toxins that trigger your immune system is what is on the end of your fork, what you inhale through your nostrils and what is in your gut." If you take care of these three crucial pathways, you will live a long and healthy life.

How many times have you said, "I can have this food/drink every once in a while, it won't hurt me." How many times have you heard "Just live a little." Here's the bottom line, each time you eat something, it harms you MUCH more than you know. The reality is, when you "live a little" you are actually "dying a little" each time. Sorry to get dark, but it's the truth. People need to stop giving themselves permission to cheat on the foods they eat. Just remember, each time you make a poor eating decision you get closer to reaching that autoimmune threshold response.

This alludes me to the primary purpose for this chapter. Wheat in any form is never going to be good for the human being. I've battled back and forth with this subject, but the research around wheat consumption in humans continues to show it is quite harmful.

The typical type of allergy testing that a person gets from an allergist is a pinprick test. This type of allergy testing is looking at immediate type hypersensitivities. In other words, it is stimulating IGE antibodies which are responsible for reactions like getting stung by a bee or exposure to peanuts. This immediate type reaction incurs from a substance called histamine.

Histamine is the reason why you will swell up and cause your skin to get red. It is the primary instigator in the inflammatory cascade. When you have too much histamine, chances are you will have systemic inflammation throughout your body. For instance, if you have always had red puffy cheeks, this probably means you've always been inflamed and you've never addressed the underlying problem. More on histamine later.

There have been studies showing the difference between Celiac wheat sensitivity and non-celiac wheat sensitivity. Celiac disease is when your body is unable to properly break down foods that contain protein called gluten in them. This can send a person's body into complete and utter destruction. I won't get into the details, but you get the point.

Researchers took people with Celiac disease and those without Celiac disease. They found when people who had Celiac were exposed to wheat products their symptoms were gastrointestinal (GI) in nature. Things like diarrhea, gas, bloating, nausea and vomiting. On the other hand, those without Celiac disease didn't express GI issues, rather they had brain dysfunction, joint disease, skin disease and fatigue.

Although the symptoms between these two groups were different, what researchers found over and over again was that each time either group ate wheat products, it ripped holes inside the lining of their intestinal tracts. IN EVERY SINGLE PARCTICIPANT. Nobody, not one single person was immune from the reaction wheat inflicted upon their digestive tract. This means that if you are a human being, when you eat wheat IT WILL DESTROY your gut lining even if you aren't having symptoms.

The reason why humans are able to inflict so much damage over time is due to how resilient our gut lining is. Our tissues covering our GI tract recover and replenish every three days. This is why we don't see awful health declines until about the age of 45. When our gut lining takes the final blow and cannot take anymore, our food particles enter through the walls of our GI tract and enter our blood stream. BAD BAD NEWS.

This is the official start of autoimmunity. Once your blood picks up food particles that have not been digested thoroughly, the body is on high alert because it perceives that food as a virus or bacteria. The immune system continually pumps out antibodies to kill the food particles repeatedly. This process continues for years until it is too late, and autoimmunity has set up a campfire with gram crackers and marshmallows.

A recent case that I heard from Dr. Thomas O'Bryan was about a three-and-a-half-year-old girl who was suffering from celiac disease. When they first diagnosed her, they went in microscopically to cut out part of her intestines to view for biopsy. It indeed turned out she had Celiac. After the procedure, however, she had a bad reaction and the doctors found she had something going on with her eye.

She was then sent out to the ophthalmologist for further workup. What they found was a conjunctival tumor, which is a tumor that typically presents as a red ball on the whites of your eyeball. Initially, they thought it was Kaposi Sarcoma which is related to HIV. This was thought to be the case because the girl's mother was HIV positive. However, the girl was HIV negative which threw a wrench in the mix. At this point, doctors decided to go forward by clipping out a piece for biopsy. The girl was then admitted to undergo surgery even though it clearly wasn't HIV related.

In the last few minutes leading up to the surgery the surgeon noticed something. He noticed that the tumor was smaller than what typically presents as Kaposi Sarcoma. He knew it wasn't Kaposi Sarcoma and just in the nick of time, the girl was saved from undergoing surgery. The next step they did with the young girl is FANTASTIC. Guess what they did?

They put this little girl on a wheat free diet with NOTHING else changed in her diet, and the conjunctival tumor went away completely. This goes to show the POWER of eliminating food products that are like bombs going off in our GI tract.

Researchers have found that if you have celiac disease it can manifest as ANYTHING and ANYWHERE in the body. It can present as cancers and autoimmune issues that cannot be explained by typical diagnosis protocols. You can live YEARS without knowing which disease or autoimmune condition you are brewing up inside, until the gates blow wide open. This is why you should ALWAYS check to see if you have a wheat sensitivity.

What the most dangerous part about Celiac disease is that researchers now show that a person has an 86 percent increase risk of dying with cardiovascular disease in the first year after being first diagnosed with Celiac disease. 86 percent!!! My oh my, that is high! This is nothing to mess around with folks.

When a person finally decides to give up wheat after consuming it for nearly their entire life, a person can expect to get sick a couple months down the line. This is because wheat contains certain kinds of prebiotics that feed our healthy gut bacteria. But, this is not the kind of prebiotics we want to feed our gut. When these people switch from wheat prebiotics to prebiotics from vegetables like asparagus and roots, the body has a tough time making such a drastic change and can leave someone sick. Don't worry though! It won't take long at all for your body to re-adapt.

Now, even some rice still has small traces of gluten in them, however they aren't nearly as harmful. If you ever do have a reaction to rice, specifically brown rice, its most likely due to a lectin sensitivity. Lectins are the proteins found on the coatings of rice and seeds as protective mechanisms from animals in the wild. That being said, typically people have less reactions to white rice. Yes, I said white rice. White rice has been given a bad name for many years because "the nutrients have been stripped away from the natural form of brown rice. Sorry to break the news, but most of the brown rice you eat isn't entirely absorbed anyhow, due to the difficulty our bodies have trying to break down brown rice compared to white rice.

Lastly, a serious condition that can spawn due to constant bombardment of wheat proteins is sepsis. Sepsis is actually a very common cause of death in the United States. Sepsis is death from bacterial infection or massive bacteria accumulation in tissues. This happens typically in the older population when their bodies become overrun with toxic bacteria. This type of bacteria that accumulates is a byproduct called Lipopolysaccharides (LPS). LPS is extremely toxic when it begins to accumulate in healthy tissues. These bacteria build up typically from a "leaky gut." LPS can take residence in your kidney, bladder, spleen, your brain and practically every organ in the body where it sees fit.

Can you now see how the integrity of your stomach and intestinal tract lining determines the quality of your life AND your skin? Can you see that autoimmunity isn't something we just get out of the blue? They are conditions that we inflict upon our OWN bodies by living a toxic and careless lifestyle. Remember what Dr. Thomas O'Bryan says, "The most common source of toxins that trigger your immune system is **what is on the end of your fork, what you inhale through your nostrils (environmental toxins) and what is in your gut**."

Autoimmune Pandemic Recap:

1. Health is not merely the absence of symptoms. You cannot claim to be healthy just because you feel good. Blood work and detailed lifestyle workups are the only predictor for absolute health.
2. Autoimmunity in the world is at an ALL TIME HIGH. At least six to seven out of ten people have autoimmune antibodies in their blood and they don't even know! This means in the coming years, symptoms will start to set in and unfortunately, they won't get the help they need from standard medical care.
3. Antibodies keep us alive and healthy. They recycle the old and damaged cells. When they are elevated this lets us know our immune system is on high alert with a high risk of autoimmunity imminent. Antibodies will then

begin to destroy health tissues of our body and send us into a spiraling decline of disease.

4. It can be years before you are officially diagnosed with autoimmunity, as doctors can't pinpoint what is going on with you. This is because symptoms are so random and minimal, they cannot properly diagnose you. You go home with a bag of medication and by the time you find your diagnosis, it's been three years and you are sicker than ever.

5. Environmental toxins (discussed later) destroy the nucleus of our cells through the stimulation of anti-nuclear antibodies. The more this occurs, our cells cannot replenish faster than they are being destroyed and the never-ending destruction continues into disease.

6. Wheat products containing gluten are always to be avoided. Plain and simple. No matter what race, color, ethnicity. If you are a HUMAN, wheat ALWAYS tears apart at your gut lining. Even if you don't feel symptoms for years to come, your digestive tract takes a beating.

Sunlight: The Generator of Life

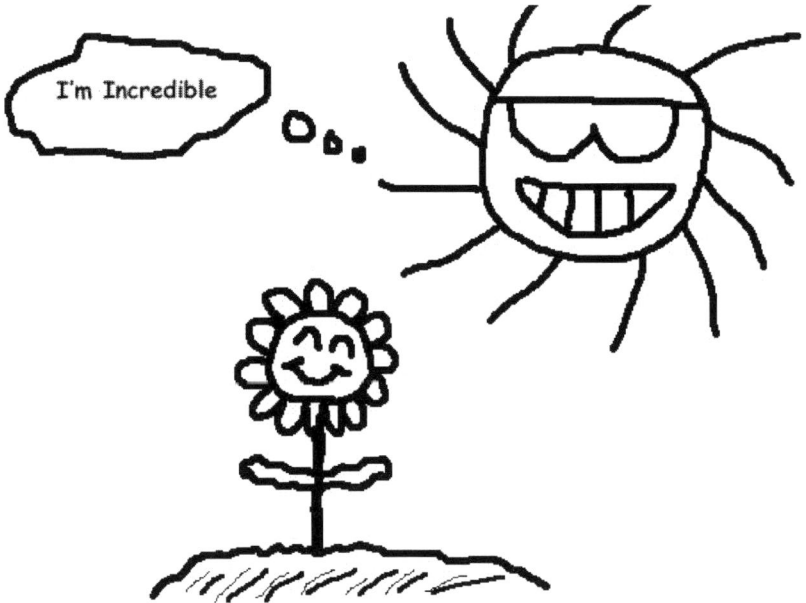

"Any patch of sunlight in a wood will show you something about the sun which you could never get from reading books on astronomy. These pure and spontaneous pleasures are 'patches of Godlight' in the woods of our experience."
— C.S. Lewis

From the dawn of time, the Earth and its habitants have been completely reliant upon the rays from the energy of our cosmic ball of light we call "The Sun." It is this ball of light that gives us day and night. Which also produces our concept of time and our 24-hour clock. In our everyday life, we disregard the sun in its existence and take much of it for granted. We forget how much of an impact it has on the organisms on Earth and throughout the cosmos. It is the sun that allows us to breathe the air that we do. Through the process of photosynthesis, all vegetation that covers Earth's soils and terrain receives its vital source of nutrition.

There is a strong emotional attachment to sunlight. Have you ever noticed how happy you feel when the sun is shining compared to a cloudy day? The sky full of a never ending blue oasis, with a slight brisk of air weaving through each arm follicle and the sun kissing every inch of your skin. It is the sun that we beg for on a frosty and chilling winter day. It is the sun we hope for when it peers just out of the clutches of a cumulonimbus cloud as we attempt to feed our skin the nutrition it oh so deserves. It is the sun that we pray for to enhance our outdoor sporting events and life experiences. And it is the sun that we thrive from to keep the entangled and complex human performing beyond all expected capability. The sun is our greatest life line. Never forget it.

Sunlight has been known for providing one of the vital ingredients our human bodies so desperately needs: Vitamin D. However, it isn't the sun that provides vitamin D. It's when sunlight reacts with human skin that it creates a cascade of events that leads to the formation of vitamin D. Now, let me clear the air before we begin. Vitamin D is not a vitamin, it is a hormone. It is when sunlight touches our skin that a cascade of events begins, and the end product is a hormone. The only reason it was named Vitamin D is from the obsession by which we believed we were deficient in it. In the profound words of my mentor Dr. Paul Goldberg, "We are not Vitamin D deficient, we are sunlight deficient." The next part will explain the pathway of hormone D. It may be boring, I know, but you'll learn something. Next time you're at a party you'll be the smartest one in the group!

Sunlight hits the skin with Ultra Violet B (UVB). UVB converts a precursor in our skin called 7-Dehydocholesterol (7DHC) into Vitamin D3 (Cholecalciferol). Vitamin D3 is then shuttled through the blood on a protein carrier to the liver. In the liver, it is converted into 25-hydroxycholecalciferol. From the liver, it travels back into the blood and arrives at the kidney. Once in the kidney it becomes the true activated form of Vitamin D which can disperse to all cells, organs, bones and tissues.

Here is the issue, many of us now take vitamin D3 supplements like candy every day. I just showed you that through this process, vitamin D3 isn't the true form of vitamin D. By using the sunlight as our source of nutrition, we have better outcomes in health and vitamin D content. Recently, there have been cases of Vitamin D3 toxicity and abuse. When you consume Vitamin D3 orally in excess, this can cause a massive buildup of calcium in the blood. This can lead to digestive distress, vomiting, nausea, fatigue, excessive thirst and frequent urination. This can also lead to kidney failure and loss of bone density when severe. However, there are some instances where supplementation is warranted and needed.

In countries that do not see sunlight often, such as northern European countries, it can be vital to get supplemental vitamin D3. Simply because sunlight is in scarcity for most of the year. Furthermore, research has shown that autoimmunity and skin conditions tend to be higher the further you move away from the equator. If you didn't already know, sunlight is the strongest and most prevalent at the equator. Which is why most populations living on or bordering the equator tend to have much darker skin pigmentation. Data shows that the further you are away from the equator, the higher incidence for autoimmune disease.

Vitamin D is so important in order for your organ systems to work properly. Vitamin D helps absorb the calcium from the food that we eat and transport that calcium into our bones. Vitamin D shuttles calcium to our heart for greater muscle contractions to eject blood more forcefully. Vitamin D is a fat-soluble hormone which is excellent for brain and cognitive health considering the brain is completely made of fat. In recent studies, researchers are considering vitamin D to be a natural nootropic. Nootropics, aka smart drugs, increase memory recall, executive functioning, cognitive enhancement and happiness.

Back to eczema. Regardless of the formation of vitamin D, direct sunlight alone is extremely valuable for you. The penetration of UVB with a wavelength of 280-315nm has been shown time and time again to be vitally imperative for the elimination of poor skin.

It is important that you adhere to strict guidelines of sun exposure, however. The sun has been demonized for fear of skin cancer in recent years. The amount of time you spend in the sun is the key for recovery. If you have darker skin, you only want to be in the sun for 20 minutes at a time on one side. Then flip over on the other side for 20 minutes. If you have very fair skin and you burn easily I highly recommend only doing 10 minutes of sunlight to begin with. The point is never to burn, as this damages your skin instead of rejuvenating it.

Do NOT, I repeat, DO NOT put on sun screen or sunblock of any kind! This is so counterproductive it blows my mind. When you put on these lotions what is it doing? It's blocking the sunlight. So, let's not do that. Contrary to what you've been told, the sun is not your enemy if you play the game correctly.

Please also know, if you didn't know already, the sun block lotions that we put on our skin are filled with carcinogens. Isn't that great? The lotion that is supposed to protect us from skin cancer is actually already promoting cancer growth before the sun even hits it! Brilliant! Have you ever stopped to think of why we ever started using sun screen? The point of sun screen is to block the sun if we plan to be outside for EXTENDED periods of time. In world we live in now, we barely step outside. 90% of our time is spent indoors now. For that reason, the pigmentation of our skin has gone from light brown to a pale white.

The pigmentation that gives us our skin color is known at melanin. When you lose melanin content, your skin becomes lighter. This can come from lack of sunlight exposure and locking yourself away from the outdoors. Thus, your skin will burn much quicker and much easier. This is why we have such a high incidence of skin cancer due to the burning of skin, leading to oxidation of tissues and perpetuation of cancer growth.

I want you to enjoy the sun. Love the sun. Embrace the sun. Do not fear it. It is one of your greatest allies in your journey to incredible skin. It will take your mood, your mind and your body to a whole other level.

My typical set up will be in a beach chair out on my driveway with my shorts rolled up all the way to my groin and the top band pulled down to my pubic area. Just letting the sun soak my face, my chest, my stomach, my legs and feet on the front side for 20 minutes. Make sure to set a timer! After 20 minutes, I flip over on the stomach and let the sun hit my entire neck, back and legs for 20 minutes. If you are a female and have access to a private location or isolated area, I recommend exposing your chest if you can. You want as much skin exposed to get maximum benefits. Again, making sure that you are not burning! We do not want any of that.

Sunlight Recap:

1. The sun has been giving light and energy to our planet for millions of years. Never take for granted the power of sunlight. It determines mood, emotion and how we perceive our day.
2. Vitamin D is vitally crucial for our existence as human beings. Without Vitamin D, we would be very sick individuals.
3. Sunlight begins the cascade of Vitamin D formation. Starting at the skin, going to the liver, then finally to the kidney where it produces true Vitamin D.
4. Consumption of Vitamin D3 is not recommended as it can lead to more harm than good. Only if you are in countries where sunlight is in scarcity should you supplement Vitamin D3.
5. Vitamin D is excellent for heart health, brain health, skin health and bone density.
6. Only expose yourself to the sun for 20 minutes at a time on each side. For a total of 40 minutes. If you have fair skin and burn easy, start out at 10 minutes max!
7. Do not apply lotion before going into the sun, for this will block the benefits of sunlight. Refrain from lotion for they typically pack harmful carcinogens.
8. Expose all skin to your comfort and appropriateness. If you can be isolated without bother, expose it all. The more, the better. But not too long! We don't want to burn!

You Only Have One Spine:
Get It Checked Regularly

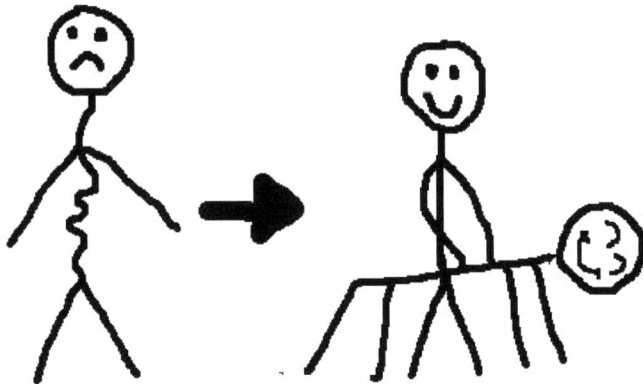

"Look well to the spine for the cause of disease."
—**Hippocrates**

You must understand that the only reason your vital organs work involuntarily is by way of your brain and spine. This is how you are able to fall asleep each night without having the fear of your heart, lungs and digestive tract failing. That is, of course, if you are without prior medical conditions such as sleep apnea. We can all agree that our brain is in control of the show, right? The brain is the master control area. The rest of our body receives information from the brain. The brain feeds directly into our spinal cord from the brain stem. From here the spinal cord runs all the way down to our tail bone (Sacrum). At each spinal level, nerve roots project out through spinal bone canals. From here these nerve roots supply the rest of our body.

These nerves serve as a neural highway of information and electrical signals that give our body energy and life. This allows us to pick up objects via muscle contractions. It allows us to use our legs and arms to voluntarily ambulate around the Earth. It allows our digestive tract to work properly and to work independently. It allows our heart to beat at regular rhythms. It allows us to give birth to children via healthy sex organs. It allows our lungs to actively expand for greater oxygen demand.

Here's the biggest mistake people make:
"I don't have back or neck pain so that means my spine must be fine. Therefore, I've never needed to see a Chiropractor."

Wrong, Wrong, Wrong!

Scenario of me asking a stranger about their spine and posture:

Me: "Have you ever been to Chiropractor?"

Them: "No, I've never needed to"

Me: "Really? Why is that?

Them: "Because I don't have neck or back pain."

Me: "Interesting. Have you ever had x-rays of your spine?"

Them: "No."

Me: "Then how can you know for certain if you have a healthy spine?"

Them: "Because I don't have pain and I just know my spine is fine."

Me: **Internal Face palm**

From here I then go into asking if they have ever had or currently have headaches, heart issues, digestion issues, breathing issues and immune dysfunction. At the end of it, I end up pulling out six or seven organ problems that they had no idea might be coming from a poor spine. Very often when we end up shooting spinal x-rays, we find there is a strong correlation with their spine and organ dysfunction.

To stress the point, a person can have ZERO PAIN but that does not mean their spine is healthy. I see it ALL the time in private practice. A person will walk in with low back pain and ZERO neck pain. However, when we take diagnostic X-rays of their neck (cervical spine), it is much worse than their lower back (lumbar spine)! When I say worse, I mean that they will have more spinal degeneration, loss of spinal disc spacing and loss of the NORMAL lordosis(curvature) of the cervical spine, while the Lumbar spine will look totally normal. When your spine is shifted away from a normal upright posture, you place excess stress onto your spinal column. When these poor postures become chronic, your muscles become weak, your bones in your spine start to degenerate and you cut off the nerve supply to your organs.

Let me ask you a question:

"Don't you think it would be pretty important to keep the nerve energy flowing to your digestive tract if you want to get rid of your Eczema and indigestion for good?"

I think YES.

The research behind poor posture and overall health has been astonishing in the last decade. When you lose the normal, natural curve in your neck this can lead to a myriad of problems. Things such neck pain, headaches, vertigo, temporomandibular joint dysfunction (TMJD), ringing in the ears, decreased immune system, visual disturbances and even decreased thyroid function can occur. These types of necks are typically referred to as "military necks" or "straight necks" when visualized on X-ray radiographs.

Poor posture not only physically harms a person via spinal health but can severely diminish a person's psychological state. Having a slumped posture, rounded shoulders and forward head posture gives way to an introvert and a poor self-image. However, it is important to know that even though a person's posture on the outside may look good, you cannot fully determine the health of a person's spine based off posture alone. A physician must take diagnostic X-rays to most accurately and precisely evaluate spinal integrity.

Through the use of X-rays, chiropractors trained in Chiropractic Biophysics® (CBP) Technique can further examine the spine by studying the curves of each spinal region based of the CBP ideal spine model. Based on your anatomy, a trained CBP doctor can determine exactly how curved your spine should be in EACH region of your spine. All Chiropractors have an EXTENSIVE amount of training in radiology (**360 HOURS** to be exact). Chiropractors are trained to detect congenital anomalies, pathological spinal processes, spinal instabilities, previous traumas/fractures and infections that all hinder spinal restoration procedures.

It is silly and naive to live a life without getting your spine checked via spinal x-rays. I recommend getting spinal x-rays at least twice per decade as a means for preventive health. And before you think getting x-rays of your spine is adding harmful radiation into your body, think again. This has been a long-time myth within the health community that has since then been proven wrong during numerous research studies. On March 10th, 2018, in the Annals of Vertebral Subluxation Research, they explain how radiogenic cancer risks from chiropractic X-rays are ZERO. Jeffrey Siegel, Ph.D. and colleagues found that radiologic imaging that was once believed to cause cancer now has no credibility and is "Fatally flawed."

You can access Annals of Vertebral Subluxation Research study here:
http://bit.ly/2FJgqX6

You can access Siegel et. Al. study here:
http://bit.ly/2GE4Xta

Food for thought: you will get MUCH more radiation from ONE trip to the airport than a single series of chiropractic x-rays.

There are **THREE** main regions of the spine:

1). Cervical Spine – This region is what makes up your neck. This region should have a LORDOTIC curve of -34 to -42 degrees with 7 moveable bones. This is the most important part of your spine. This is where the Brain first connects to the spinal cord. All information flows first through the neck before it can get to the rest of the body. Thus, if you don't first have a healthy cervical spine, you cannot be your healthiest self. This also means your digestive tract won't get as much energy as it would if you had a healthy cervical spine first.

Common conditions associated with Cervical spine dysfunction:
- Neck Pain
- Shoulder Pain
- Numbness and Tingling in Hands and Fingers
- Weakness in Hands/Grip Strength
- Sinusitis
- Chronic Allergies
- Cold Hands
- Headaches
- Vertigo
- Dizziness
- Nausea
- Fatigue/Lethargy
- Depression/Poor Self Image
- Temporomandibular Joint Dysfunction (TMJD – pain and clicking in jaw)
- Grinding Teeth at Night
- Ringing in The Ears
- Decreased immune system (getting sick easier and staying sick longer than most people)
- Visual disturbances (floaters, flashing lights, blurred vision)
- Decreased thyroid function

2). Thoracic spine – This region of your spine makes up your upper back and middle back. This region should have a KYPHOTIC curve of -44 degrees with 12 moveable bones. This is part of the spine controls the heart, lungs, stomach, small intestine, kidneys, gall bladder, spleen and pancreas. BINGO. The **THORACIC** and **LUMBAR** spine are the biggest areas of concern with digestive issues considering this is where all digestive organs reside. We want to make sure our spine and posture is pristine in these areas to eliminate all chance of organ dysfunction.

Common conditions associated with Thoracic spine dysfunction:
- Heart Murmurs
- Heart Palpitations
- Fast/slow Beating Heart
- High/low Blood Pressure
- Heart Attacks/Heart Pains
- Shortness of Breath
- Asthma/Wheezing
- Recurrent Lung Infections
- Pain on Deep Inspiration/Expiration
- Pain in Ribs
- Blood Sugar Dysfunction/Diabetes
- Indigestion
- Heart Burn
- Acid Reflux
- Stomach Ulcers

3). Lumbar spine – This region makes up your lower back. This region should have a LORDOTIC curve of -40 degrees with 5 moveable bones. This area of the spine controls the large intestine, sex organs, prostate, bladder and uterus. This is important because if you are also suffering with inflammatory bowel disease such as Crohn's disease or ulcerative colitis, your lumbar spine could be at play.

Common conditions associated with Lumbar spine dysfunction:
- Low Back Pain
- Hip and Leg Pain
- Weakness in Legs and Feet
- Leg Cramps
- Coldness in Legs and Feet
- Numbness and Tingling in Feet/Toes
- Frequent/Painful/Difficult Urination
- Constipation/Diarrhea
- Gas/Bloating

- Crohn's Disease and Ulcerative Colitis
- Bladder Infections
- Heavy Bleeding/Cramping During Menstrual Cycles
- Sexual Dysfunction, Loss of Sex Drive, Difficulties Conceiving (Quite Common!)

REMEMBER:

Your skin is reflective upon the health and functioning of your DIGESTIVE TRACT. The nerves from your Thoracic and Lumbar spine directly supply your digestive tract. If your spine is out of proper alignment, there is a high chance those same nerves are unhealthy and will affect your ability to process foods. This means your food WILL NOT be broken down as effectively and nutrients WILL NOT be sent to the vital cells and tissues of your body. Thus, inflammation sets in, food particles will find their way into your blood stream and your immune system will be on high alert as if your food is an invader. This will cause systemic stress which shows itself on YOUR SKIN.

Go visit a doctor who SPECIALIZES in Spinal Corrective Care without the use of drugs and surgery. Also known as Chiropractors. To make it easier for you to find a doctor in your area visit the Ideal Spine Doctor Directory:

https://idealspine.com/directory/

You can enter your zip code and see who the closest Chiropractic Biophysics (CBP) Doctor is nearest you!

Your Spine Health Recap:

1. Our brain plugs directly into our spinal cord. Our spinal cord then runs down all of our spinal bones. If our spinal bones are shifted out of place. It can affect the nerves leaving the spinal cord. This can put stress on your ENTIRE body and digestive tract! Thus, rendering your stomach and intestines weaker with the inability to break down foods properly.

2. You CAN have a poor spine and posture without ANY pain. This means you should definitely get your spine checked through diagnostic x-rays for preventive measures. You could be suffering from a massive spinal distortion that is affecting your overall health, but you have zero signs or symptoms. If you want, I will personally look at your x-rays.

3. There are three regions of the spine. Cervical, Thoracic and Lumbar. Each are just as important as the next. One area can shift out of place and affect another area. Meaning, your spine is a constantly moving and an ever-shifting dynamic entity. It has ebbs and flows. The spine is a UNIT. Take care of it as such.

4. Get your spine checked by a Chiropractor who specializes in Advanced Spinal Rehabilitation at Idealspine.com under the doctor directory. Reach out to me if you need help finding a provider in your area.

The Boogeyman:
Environmental Toxins

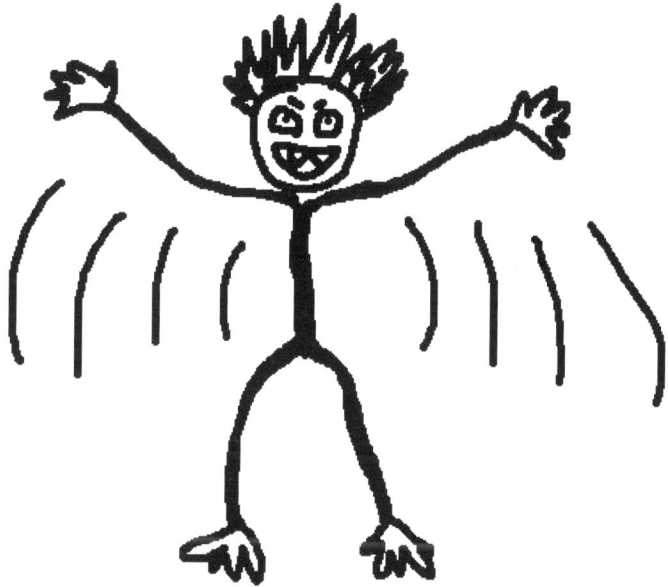

"One man's poison ivy is another man's spinach"
-George Ade

Now, there are MANY environmental toxins that most people are already aware of. Things like carbon monoxide, radon gases, BPA in plastics, estrogen in the water supply from flushing tampons and the list goes on. We could be here all day if you left me to talk about these poisons, but I won't do that to you. However, there are two toxins that hide from plain sight and are not talked about enough. These are the things I want to bring to the surface. They could be adding to your inability to get the results you are looking for. Remember, the human body is very sensitive. Each person responds differently to their environment. For instance, my father and I are very allergic to cat dander, whereas my mother and brother are totally immune. The idea of human individuality has been lost in our current paradigm of health care today. It is through this book that I hope to reinstate your understanding of how unique you are compared to everyone around you.

First: **MOLD TOXINS**

Would it be okay if I first start off by sharing my personal experience with toxic mold exposure? It will certainly set the stage for what is to come. When I was in undergraduate school at the University of Florida in Gainesville, Florida, I lived in a decently old and weathered house. Now, I don't know if you are a sports fan or not, but the football stadium for the Florida Gators is nick named "The Swamp." The first reason should be obvious, as alligators live in swamps all over Florida. The second is when you play football in the state of Florida or any other sport for that matter, it is extremely hot and muggy almost year-round. That being said, it is as if the entire state of Florida is a swamp and its residents are living in its humid, wet and soggy weather every day.

Not only does this climate affect the outdoor life of Florida, but it also immediately affects the housing and ventilation within

Florida homes. It is very easy for the humidity to start ripping away at the wood infrastructure and air conditioning systems. When water is trapped in an area where it cannot escape, where there is no light, where there is no heat or wind to dry the moisture up, it begins to collect bacteria. Thus, mold is born. Not only does it stay within the confines of its original settlement, but it becomes airborne through our air conditioning vents. This is when you get into big trouble.

Since my house had been a seasoned piece of property, you could almost predict with 100% certainty it had either water damage and mold growing. What is worse, the house was almost completely covered by a massive oak tree and tall pine trees in the surrounding area. Thus, not much sunlight was able to penetrate through the windows, which left most of the house damp and dark. When you walked into the house, you could actually smell the mustiness in the air. The house had wooden floors that would creak and crack as you walked across the boards. There was apparent water damage, all you had to do is look up at the ceiling. But, being a poor undergraduate student, I was only worried about being close to campus and paying the least amount for rent. This taught me a VALUABLE lesson – Your HEALTH is worth more than all the money in the world. Don't sacrifice your health just to save a couple of dollars.

Now, being a young adult, I also was ignorant of the potential health risks living in that home. I also had no idea that any of the water damage really mattered. The WORST part of the house was in my bathroom. It turns out that I had been showering in a bathroom that had A MASSIVE amount of black mold covering the entire ceiling. I want to add that the water in that shower got extremely hot and the bathroom steamed up significantly during each shower. Unknowingly, this steam was rising up into the ceiling and the toxic black mold was releasing spores into my mouth and nose. It wasn't until my cousin came to visit for my graduation that he told me I had a very bad mold infestation.

I had been living in this house for two years and had never once thought that my health issues were coming from the mold toxins. I never once had eczema until I lived in that house. And I didn't have cloudy thoughts, lethargy and neurological imbalances until I moved into that house. It was at this point that everything came full circle. My way of living and the environment around me had become the reason my health was declining at a rapid rate. By working out seven days a week, taking pre-workout drinks and toxic protein powders every day, staying up way too late and living in a home with mold toxins, my internal organs and body were being CRUSHED.

Now, you may not have immediate symptoms from mold exposure, but long-term exposure can have detrimental effects on your ENTIRE health. You may not even know you are inhaling mold spores through your air conditioning system. However, if you live in a humid climate, getting your ventilation systems cleaned is a MUST. Considering that humans now live 90% of their lives indoors, it is imperative that you get your air quality examined. Indoor circulating air is now much more toxic than outdoor air.

Symptoms from mold exposure could be things that have now become a part of your life. Things such as:

- Chronic Allergies and Sinusitis
- Getting Sick Easier and Staying Sick Longer Than Most People (Decreased Immune System)
- Chronic Respiratory Infections
- Chronic Coughs/Wheezing/Asthma
- Shortness of Breath
- Brain Fog/Confusion
- Memory Loss/Learning Disorders
- Dizziness
- Headaches
- Lethargy/Chronic Fatigue/Sleep Disorders
- Depression/Personality Disorders
- Dry, Scaly and Itchy Skin (ECZEMA)

If you take anything away from this, KNOW that black mold is EXTREMELY NEUROTOXIC. Meaning that it affects your BRAIN and NERVOUS SYSTEM almost immediately. This literally means brain and nerve cells are being killed each time you are exposed to this mold. This not only affects your cognitive and processing power but also affects THE ENTIRE rest of your body systems. If your body is continually stressed by an immune system disruptor (mold), then your body will remain in a state of inflammation and high alert. This will decrease your ability to break down foods, eliminate waste products, diffuse clean oxygen through lung tissue and the ability for your immune system to fight intruders (meaning you are sick more often). This is when you will start to see your skin respond with eruptions, scales, pustules, patches and red splotches.

I had Eczema EVERYWHERE. Under my eyes, my forehead, ears, armpits, forearms, PRIVATE PARTS, butt cheeks, thighs, calves, toes and back. At first, I used corticosteroid creams for temporary relief, but it KEPT coming back. I thought I just needed to shower more and apply topical ointments like coconut oil. Nothing worked. Even looking into supplements to help, yup that also failed. Its alarming how misunderstood skin conditions are by the medical community (dermatologists) and even by self-proclaimed health gurus who dispense supplements like drug reps. When did we get so detached from eating things from the Earth and enjoying the great outdoors? The more we get away from Earth's soil, the sicker we seem to become.

Your skin is the largest organ of the body. It is the last organ to reveal signs of health or disease. This means that when you see pimples, eczema, psoriasis, and other skin disorders, your internal body has already been fighting battles before it shows up on your skin. Your skin can be thought of as the lighthouse sending out beacons of light to let you know where your current state of health is at. You must understand, that having any kind of skin blemish, bump, irritation and eruption is not normal. It is mind boggling that kids who grow up with pimples accept that "It's just puberty." How about doctors check to see what they are eating, what their current environmental setting is, their stress levels? Then do further workups through blood testing of food allergies. Instead, we turn immediately to topical ointments and oral medications that make the conditions much worse.

Second: **Electromagnetic Frequencies (EMF)**

We now live in the technological age where every single human has a cellphone in their pocket. We have routers and modems in almost every home. We actually place our laptops on our LAPS. We have smart tablets for our entertainment needs. We have blue tooth and wireless headphones plugging right into our ears. We have powerlines so close, they are practically on top of our houses. We place cellphones right up to our faces when talking on the phones, which is like gluing a microwave oven to our head. While on the subject, we also use microwaves to heat up our foods, not to mention the radiation given off by these devices. Oh, and how microwaves conveniently heat up our foods but also completely mutate the DNA and proteins of our foods. Which, quite frankly, turn our foods into immediate "Franken-foods."

The point of the matter is that our bodies are being OVERLOADED with radiation doses not tolerated well by any animal, creature and living entity on planet Earth. Just as mold toxins are "out of sight out of mind," EMF toxicity is of grave concern recently. Humans don't believe there is much to EMFs simply because they cannot physically see the rays of radiation. However, the amount of EMF today is affecting how we sleep, reproduce, behave and think in our everyday life. If you live in an apartment, chances are you are receiving radiation from up to 10 different neighbors around you, which is a significant amount. EMF exposure directly impacts the cells of your body. Most importantly, the cells of your mitochondria which are directly involved with your ENERGY PRODUCTION. Long term exposure can mutate and distort normal functioning cells into irregular and unusable cells. Overtime these cells can become malignant and have the potential to turn into more sinister cancer cells.

The ability for a woman to become pregnant in today's age is getting much more difficult. The reproductive organs of both male and female counterparts are EXTREMELY sensitive to ionizing radiation. Recent studies have shown the detrimental impact EMF has on sexual reproduction. Men and women all over are wondering why they cannot have a baby and the answer to their sterility is simple: Limit the amount of EMF around their private parts. This means whenever you put your cell phone into your pocket, turn it on airplane mode, as this will cut all signals coming from the phone. It may seem like a daunting task at first, but it becomes second nature quickly.

You must ask yourself: Do you want to suffer the risk of not having kids and genitourinary malignancies or would you rather stay away from your crack phone? This goes the same for laptops. NEVER EVER place your laptop on your LAP! The regulations in the United States for EMF output on cellular devices, laptops and other wireless devices have an almost unlimited amount of radiation output. The European Nations understand the harm of EMF from wireless devices and have very strict regulations on previously stated devices.

Studies have explained that EMF exposure affects the nervous system directly. This means anything controlled by the nervous system is indirectly affected. So essentially, the entire body is being harmed. More importantly is the endocrine system, responsible for hormone production and fertility. Researchers studied the affect EMF had on the neuroendocrine system (nervous system + endocrine system) and what they found didn't surprise them much. They found that EMF induced cell death in testicular germ cells in mice, a decrease in serum testosterone and decrease sperm production. In women, researchers believe EMF accelerates the process of apoptosis (programmed cell death) in the ovaries and leads to death of ovarian cortical tissue and cells in the uterus and fallopian tubes.

There are many other physiology conditions currently associated with EMF exposure:
- Cell Replication Disorders
- DNA Damage
- Chromosomal Abnormalities
- Blood Disorders (BIG FOR ECZEMA)
- Birth Defects
- Hormone Production Dysfunction
- Respiratory Distress and Dysfunction

A declassified report showed that military personnel exposed to non-thermal microwave radiation experienced:
- Headaches
- Fatigue
- Dizziness
- Irritability
- Sleeplessness
- Depression
- Forgetfulness
- Lack of Concentration

(Havas Magda. Engineering and Technology History. 1976. Biological Effects of Electromagnetic Radiation.)

Just to recap – EMF does quite a bit of harm to all the cells of the body, even if it isn't immediately apparent. One person may be much more sensitive to EMFs and will experience symptoms. While others may not feel one bit of discomfort. This DOES NOT mean it isn't equally affecting both people. This goes the same for mold toxins.

Realistically speaking, you cannot escape the exposure of EMF unless you live out in a farmland, plain or forested area. This I know. However, you CAN make sure you aren't adding any insult to injury. This means when you place your cellphone in your pocket to put it on airplane mode. When you are using your laptop place it on a table or desk – anywhere except your lap. THROW YOUR MICROWAVE OUTSIDE AND BEAT IT WITH A BASEBALL BAT. Stop being lazy. Heat up your food in the oven, stovetop or convection oven. Take the extra time to make sure what you are eating isn't being turned into some weird denatured food product. If you have a router place it far away from your room because wireless routers/modems DO AFFECT your sleep patterns and rhythms. This also goes for your cell phone – place it on airplane mode next to your bed. Sleep is more important than getting a late-night text anyhow. If you are living next to or near a powerline, you really NEED to move. I can't even express how much this is going to eat away at your cells and overall health.

Going back to human individuality. Everyone in the world is different when it comes to being allergic or hypersensitive to environmental toxins. No two people are alike, unless they are twins. Even now researchers are finding small differences in gene comparisons in twins. You see, twins might be born genetically identical but the way they decide to live their life will either enhance or degrade their DNA. This is a field known at epigenetics. Meaning that whatever genes you are born with can be changed based on the health decisions and choices you make in your life. For instance, if you were born with genes linked to a greater risk of developing cancer, this DOES NOT mean you will get cancer. Genes coding for various diseases are turned ON when you make poor life choices such as drinking, smoking, chronic stress, recreational drugs, chronic exposure to toxic chemicals/irritants, eating foods with pesticides, added hormones and genetically modified organisms. This means YOU ARE NOT a prisoner of your unfortunate family lineage! You are the driver of your health and well-being! You also shape the health of your offspring. So, choose now and choose wisely. For you ACTUALLY have a say in the matter for the future of your family tree. More on epigenetics next.

Environmental Toxins Recap:
1. Mold growth can be anywhere without you taking notice to it until you start developing health conditions that seem to come from nowhere.
2. Mold is neurotoxic and can severely destroy brain cells. This leads to memory impairment, increased risk for dementia and depression.
3. What affects our brain will also severely impact the rest of our body.
4. Electromagnetic Radiation is almost inescapable in our technological driven world. However, you have the power to limit the amount you are exposed to
5. Our cell phones, laptops, TVs, microwaves, Bluetooth devices are the biggest producers of EMF radiation. We can limit the amount of EMF we bombard our body's most vital cells with switching phones into airplane mode, getting rid of microwave ovens and limiting the time we put laptops on our LAPS.

Epigenetics: Control Your Present and Future

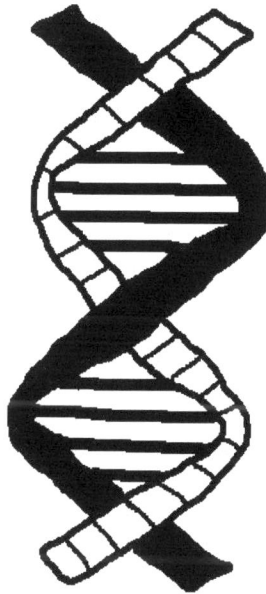

"Take care of your body. It's the only place you have to live."
-Jim Rohn

Good news! You get to decide the fate of your life. You get to decide how long you want to live. You get to decide how healthy you can be. Do you want to know how? It's this little-known field called Epigenetics. You see... people think they are stuck with the genes they were born with. Well, technically you are stuck with your family genes. However, YOU get to decide if you turn those genes on or off. Many diseases that pose a strong familial connection can lay dormant for your entire life! The chances of you acquiring various autoimmunity diseases can be passed down from your parents but it is up to you to express those genes!

The way you eat, sleep, and interact ALL play a huge role in how your genes will be expressed when you pass it down to your offspring. For example, if your whole life you were into working out and eating healthy, chances are your child will be a thoroughbred. This is why you may have a friend who is just naturally ripped or in shape all the time, even though they eat garbage foods. This is also why these people are able to lose weight and build muscle much faster than the average person. It is no secret that genes play a massive role in how a person's life will turn out. But you must realize you have the power to shape not only your future but the rest of your family lineage by just living to your full potential.

Another example on the opposite side of the spectrum are the people who have a tough time losing weight. It's not that these people haven't tried to lose weight through many avenues, it is just that they have a harder time losing weight and takes much longer. When it takes two or three times longer than the average person to lose weight, these people become discouraged and give up. Once they throw in the towel, they put on weight much quicker than average people. It also doesn't help that the majority of these people typically grow up in an environment where their parents don't exactly live a healthy lifestyle. Monkey see, monkey do.

This all goes to say, PEOPLE ARE BUILT DIFFERENTLY. More specifically, some people are just more sensitive to certain foods, environmental toxins/allergens and stress. Everyone has their own health story. If you dive deep into ANY person's life, they at one point either had or HAVE a health problem or concern. It is impossible to live a life completely devoid of sickness or ailment that needs careful tending to. So just remember, when you think you are the only one with Eczema or any disorder for that matter, you are far from alone. Unfortunately, some people wait too long to make a drastic step in their health NOW and suffer debilitating diseases later.

I don't think I need to beat the dead horse repeatedly to get you to believe Epigenetics is what makes us unique. But I'll do it anyway. Epigenetics is why some of us have blonde, brown or black hair. It is why some of us are White, Black, Asian or Latino. It is why some of us HATE sea food, but love land meats. Ever wondered why you really hated a food when you were young but loved it as you got older? Yep, your genes gave you what we call an "acquired taste" although we typically express this phrase as an unpopular food choice.

Newer research has shown that a mother's exposure to environmental toxins could impact her child's susceptibility to autoimmune diseases. Most of our society focuses on the mother while she is pregnant. For a mother to avoid smoking and drinking alcohol is a no brainer that everyone is aware of. However, it doesn't just stop with the mother's contribution. Studies have recently shown that a child's mental ability could be influenced by the father's diet.

Studies in mice revealed that fathers who had a diet rich in folic acid and vitamin B12 gave birth to offspring who had slower cognitive functioning and slower memory recall. Now, this might be a stretch for you to believe, but if you were born with slower than normal brain functioning, this could very well affect the rest of your body. INCLUDING your digestion and how your skin presents itself.

Now, epigenetic traits are more stable within adulthood but are still VERY MUCH modifiable. Our environment (the air we breathe) has become a big problem as of late, with a strong correlation with neurodegenerative diseases like Alzheimer's and Dementia. Without a doubt, the biggest player in how your genes are shaped and modified comes FROM WHAT YOU EAT. The field of nutri-epigenomics studies how food and your genes work together to influence your longevity on planet Earth. Although the Ketogenic diet currently is excessively talked about, studies consistently show this type of diet is extremely conducive to a healthy lifestyle. For those of you who don't know what a Ketogenic diet is, it is a diet composed of healthy fats, adequate protein and low amounts of carbohydrates in the form of vegetable carbohydrates.

Quickly, without completely boring you, I'm going to cover the technical side of epigenetics for the analytical reader. Just about every single disease that has a strong hereditary correlation is determined by this concept of DNA METHYLATION. All you need to know is that Methyl (CH_3) groups are groups of one carbon with 3 hydrogens attached to it. These methyl groups are attached to DNA which can modify your genes and affect how certain traits like eye and skin color. When you have too many or too little of these methyl groups for selected gene, this can perpetuate diseases in a once healthy human being. Those who already carry the gene, let's say cancer, are much more likely to express that gene if they choose to smoke, eat poorly, drink too much alcohol and have toxic relationships, etc.

There are many diseases related to either hypo (little) and hyper(many) methylation. People with hyper-methylation can suffer from diseases such as schizophrenia, bipolar illnesses, and psychosis. Whereas those with hypo-methylation can suffer from autoimmune conditions such as lupus. It is also important to note that many other autoimmune conditions play a role in how healthy your digestion can be. Conditions like ulcerative colitis, Crohn's and Celiac disease can all very well be related to hypo-methylation. It is important and relieving to know that our genes are always in state of flux. Always changing and adapting.

It is important to note that our gut flora (our natural gut bacteria) are the only reason we are able to live and breathe on this planet. They are the reason we can break down foods and shuttle those nutrients to the cells of our body. They can literally affect our emotional state, our cognitive performance and overall health depending on the current health of those colonies. The reason I speak about this is mainly because recent research has shown that our gut flora can be changed very rapidly in response to dietary changes. Which are directly related to microbial GENE EXPRESSION. These studies even show the relation to the health of the gut microbiome and your chances of acquired Crohn's disease aka inflammatory bowel disease.

A LARGE amount of evidence reveals that children exposed to more bacteria from animals, molds, pollens and dirt debris are MUCH less likely to suffer from allergies/autoimmunity compared to those children who live in squeaky clean environments. You see, we NEED bacteria from the Earth and should refrain from over-sanitizing everything. I mean, it makes sense, right? We LIVED off the Earth for THOUSANDS of years. We belong to the soils of Earth, not the soils of tile floors, wooden floors and carpets that are cleaned by a maid service once a week. Our immune systems are now very weak because we have no outside intruder to test our immune system. Therefore, our immune system lays dormant, taking an overextended vacation, when out of nowhere it is attacked, caught off guard. This is when autoimmunity starts sneaking its way in.

The primary reason for me writing this chapter in the book is to say YOU ARE DIFFERENT. YOU ARE UNIQUE. YOU ARE NOT LIKE

ANYONE ELSE ON PLANET EARTH. Can you start to see how repetitive I get? There is a reason I am repetitive. It is to ENGRAIN this concept into your brain! If you only walk away with learning one thing from this book it is that YOU ARE AN INDIVIDUAL WITH INDIVIDUAL NEEDS.

The most likely reason you have Eczema is from your over-sensitivity to either things you eat or the things you breathe in. When you adopt a lifestyle that fits your needs, you WILL NOT have Eczema breakouts. If this means you must cut back on drinking alcohol and coffee so be it. If this means you must give up dairy and gluten so be it. If you are having Eczema outbreaks, what do you think is happening on the inside? Answer – Utter Chaos.

Each day you continue to let Eczema ruin your life or cover Eczema up by using corticosteroid creams, is another day you let your body proceed toward disease and decay. It sounds dark, I know, but it is reality. You are quite literally mutating your genes each day you let your Eczema continue to perpetuate. Not to mention, by adding harmful corticosteroid creams into your body. Man, those are nasty creams. If you could only be a fly on the wall inside your body, you would shut down this operation immediately.

I highly recommend getting a comprehensive food allergy and environmental allergy panel. Best lab testing comes from BLOOD in my opinion. I would also highly suggest ordering a 23andMe Ancestry+Health panel. It is fairly inexpensive considering they do a full ancestry panel and health panel to see which diseases you are at risk for based off your genes. It's certainly worth the investment to know. It will tell you things like if you carry the APOE gene for Alzheimer's, lactose intolerance, genetic weight loss issues, gut and digestive issues and many more.

The bottom line is this: You get to shape the health of your life through how you live. What you decide to put in your mouth either has consequences or benefits. The environment you chose to hang around determines the quality of air you decide to feed your lungs and blood cells. The relationships you create are either blossoming or they are broken. Our emotional status drives a large amount of our overall well-being through healthy hormone cycling. Increased cortisol (stress hormone) production in our body contributes to disruption of normal DNA methylation, which leads to poor gene regulation. Translation: our genes we acquired from our lineage that are associated with disease are LITERALLY being flipped on JUST FROM EMOTIONAL DISTRESS ALONE!

Now can you see how miniscule lifestyle changes can make a WORLD of difference in the realm of youth, vitality and happiness? It isn't rocket science. The simple things that make us function as humans based off our genome have always been right there in front of us. We just choose to live beyond what our bodies were designed for. Is it a surprise to you that when we consume toxins that our body refuses it? Is it so hard to understand that in order to be healthy, you must give up the things your body is telling you EVERY DAY to stop? Things like drinking alcohol, smoking tobacco and eating highly processed foods are some of the vices that we should have never been exposed to. However, we are humans and whenever we receive or consume something that rewards us with immediate satisfaction we cannot help ourselves. If it were one flaw humans have, it is that we desire and crave more than our physiology and biology can handle.

If you take care of your body, your genes will take care of you. Remember, you can be stuck with the burden of having poor genes, BUT YOU GET TO DECIDE if they turn on or not! You also get to decide if you want to change your genes and pass them off to your offspring and lineage to come! You may have trouble adapting to a life that is well suited for your genes at first, but once you understand what your body NEEDS and DESIRES, your body will start working for YOU! You will no longer feel tired, groggy, unhappy and sick. Your energy levels will skyrocket. Your personal relationships will flourish. Your sleep will be impeccable. Your digestion will be pristine. And, Oh yea... YOUR SKIN WILL LOOK AMAZING!

Be good to your genes and they will provide unlimited power and potential for all of your years on this planet!

Epigenetics Recap:

1. Your genes do not determine your future health. YOU determine your lifespan and happiness by the decisions you make by investing in your health from all angles.
2. Epigenetics is what makes us unique. It is what determines which environmental allergens and foods we tolerate and do not tolerate.
3. The way you choose to live your life will determine the fate of your family lineage. If you've worked out your entire life, chances are your child will have "fit" genetics.
4. What you eat, what you breathe, where you hang out and who you choose to hang out with can readily modify your unique genetics.
5. Genetic modification is driven by DNA methylation and is directly correlated with the inheritance of certain familial diseases. You decide if your family genes kill you or not... just saying.
6. Gene expression is strongly related to the health of our gut. Depending on the health of our beneficial gut bacteria, this can rapidly change our genome, plus the emotional and physical state of our health.
7. Children exposed to as much natural bacteria from mud, molds, dirt and grasses are less likely to have any allergies or digestive sensitivities later in their life.
8. Get allergy and genetic panels to see exactly what your body rejects and accepts. It is worth it and takes out the guess work. Make the investment.

9. Your genes are more and more likely to determine your fate. But it is up to you to nurture them to your advantage. Stop making it difficult. Get to know your body. It will treat your right if you do.

Histamine: Inflammation Gone Wild

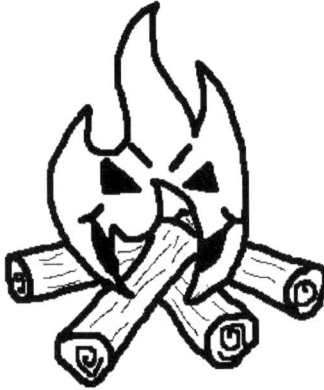

"Life expectancy would grow by leaps and bounds if green vegetables smelled as good as bacon."
-Doug Larson

If you have been struggling with Eczema for some time now, you are no stranger to the word "inflammation." You have most likely heard of diets that try to reduce inflammation AT ALL COST. Diets that consist of a plethora of supplements designed to eliminate the amount of systemic inflammation you have endured over the years. While I don't disagree with some of the methods with these diets, I do think the craze of killing inflammation completely has become a little excessive. Here is why...

We NEED inflammation to occur in our bodies. Inflammation is the only way we are able to recover from bruises, cuts and injuries. For example, if you suffer a blow to your leg you will notice a large amount of swelling with black and blue discoloration that we call bruising. This bruising is from the massive amount of blood that has been shuttled to the site of injury. When your body suffers an injury it immediately responds with excess blood supply to that area, so it can send clotting factors and chemical messengers to repair the area of concern. This is when histamine comes into play.

Histamine is chemical messenger involved in the normal inflammation pathway. When our tissues(skin) becomes damaged, mast cells in our skin release this chemical histamine. Histamine then triggers the dilation of our blood vessels (making our blood vessels expand) so more blood can be flooded to the site of injury. The blood vessels bring in large amounts of clotting factors that are responsible to make sure we don't bleed to death. White blood cells then show up and clean up and eat the damaged tissues. You see, without histamine we would never be able to heal from injury. When the histamine response is normal, it is extremely beneficial. But when it is over produced, it can be a recipe for disaster.

Histamine is also involved in our normal allergen responses. Things like runny nose, itchy eyes, hives, decreased breathing. This is why when you are allergic to the changing seasons or having an animal allergy you take anti-histamines to decrease the over-reaction of histamine. The problem with doing this, is that you are suppressing the ability for your body to warn you that you are in danger. Although it will suppress your symptoms, your body is still being damaged by the environmental allergen.

Histamine intolerance is a fairly new condition in the health field today when related to diet and lifestyle. Researchers are not exactly certain why some people have an overabundance of histamine in their bodies. The top three theories at the moment point to genetics, enzyme deficiency and DNA methylation abnormalities.

Though more studies must be done, there is a genetic component to histamine intolerance. Others may have enzymatic dysfunction with having lower than normal amounts of Diamine Oxidase (DAO) which is primarily responsible for the breakdown of circulating histamine. Lastly, others may produce too much histamine by having too much Histidine Decarboxylase which is the enzyme responsible for changing histidine (amino acid) into histamine usually from DNA methylation dysfunction.

Of importance, histamine intolerance has a strong correlation with the health of a person's gut. There are certain bacteria that produce histamine and if these bacteria are dominating the gut flora, histamine could be circulating out of control. It is important to note that most people with histamine intolerance are nutrient deficient because they typically have a leaky gut as well. Histamine enzymes are created in our guts and when our gut is unhealthy it is unable to produce the enzymes needed to breakdown histamine.

It is important to FIRST fix any digestive dysfunction before you can fix histamine intolerance. However, people will find that trying to use natural probiotics like fermented foods to heal their gut will actually make it worse. As I list below, fermented foods create a massive histamine response. Therefore, one should supplement a bacterial strain like Bifidobacterium BASED OFF THEIR

STOOL TEST! Do not blindly pick up a probiotic thinking it will help you.

You can get blood tests to check for histamine levels and Diamine Oxidase levels. This will test your ratio of histamine/DAO. If you have a high ratio histamine/DAO, this means you are eating too much histamine and you don't have enough DAO to break down histamine.

You may also get the integrity of your gut lining tested through Zonulin and LPS labs. Zonulin is what controls the tight junctions inside your gut lining. In other words, it controls what goes through your gut wall and what does not.

LPS (lipopolysaccharide) testing can reveal if you have leaky gut or not. If LPS levels are high, it means your immune system is currently fighting an overload of bacteria.

These tests are important to see where you stand in your overall health. If you would like me to special order these for you, please let me know.

Common Causes of Histamine Intolerance:

- Small Intestinal Bacterial Overgrowth (SIBO)
- Leaky gut
- Fermented foods, drinks and alcohols
- Diamine Oxidase deficiency
- Immediate type allergies (pollens, animals, bee stings)
- Eating histamine-rich foods

Causes of Low Diamine Oxidase:

- Small Intestinal Bacterial Overgrowth (SIBO)
- Inflammatory bowel disease (Crohn's, Ulcerative Colitis)
- Gluten Intolerance
- Leaky Gut
- Alcohol, Energy Drinks, Tea
- Medications:
  Antihistamines, Immunosuppressants, Antidepressants,
  Antacids, Antiarrhythmics, NSAIDS.

HIGH Histamine Foods to Avoid:

- ALL fermented foods (sauerkraut, pickles, kimchi, vinegar, soy sauce, yogurt)
- Aged cheeses (even though you shouldn't eat dairy anyhow)
- Smoked meats
- Shellfish
- Beans OF ALL KINDS (peanuts, black, soy, pinto, chickpeas)
- Nuts – Walnuts, Cashews, Peanuts
- Chocolate
- Vinegars (pickles, mayonnaise, olives)
- Canned meats and ready to eat meals
- Any packaged foods with preservatives and artificial colorings
- Tomatoes, Papaya, Pineapple, Strawberries, Bananas, Avocados, Spinach, Eggplant, Mushroom and Dried Fruit, Citrus Fruits
- LEFTOVER MEALS (aged foods can increase histamine formation)
- Wheat germ
- Yeasts
- Soy products
- Peas

HIGH Histamine Drinks to Avoid:

- ALL alcoholic beverages (beer, wine, champagne etc.)
- Fermented drinks – kombucha, kefir (water and milk)
- Teas
- Coffee
- Energy Drinks
- Cow's Milk

LOW Histamine Foods and Drinks:

- Fresh organic meats (beef, chicken, uncured pork, turkey)
- Freshly caught fish (wild)
- Whole eggs (cooked)
- Fresh fruits (other than those listed above)
- Gluten free grains: Rice
- Fresh vegetables (previous page)
- Dairy substitutes: coconut milk, almond milk
- Cooking oils: olive oil, coconut oil

It is important to also recognize that when you are stressed, mast cells release histamine in your tissues. If you are chronically stressed from work, relationships and even during your healing process your ability to get better will be diminished by the flooding of histamine in your body. Doing breathing drills, journaling and meditation as I mentioned earlier in the book will help with the stress response. Now are you starting to see how everything I am teaching you is starting to come full circle? Instead of thinking of a magic pill or potion, you must figure out what works for YOU.

Here is the thing. You must not freak out and avoid all of these foods just because I mentioned you might POSSIBLY have a reaction to histamine. The only way to KNOW for CERTAIN if you have a reaction to histamine is to TEST TEST TEST! The guessing game is what got you into this mess to begin with. Please do not treat this as another one of your failed Dr. Google attempts where you blindly accept online information as fact. I DO NOT want you to always take info that you learn as fact. Always question what you learn. Be a scientist. Do self-experiments. More importantly, DO BLOOD TESTING! Your blood never lies. It will always tell you what you lack, what you have too much of and if you are within normal limits. Investments in lab testing NOW, will save you THOUSANDS in healthcare later. Just get them done!

Treat your gut with care, stabilize your histamine response, enhance your life.

IN THAT ORDER ☺

Histamine Recap:
1. Histamine is a vital chemical messenger needed during a normal inflammatory response during injury or infection.
2. Abnormal levels of Histamine can lead to increased allergic response to food and environmental pollens/toxins.
3. There are three main theories why histamine levels rise: genetic inheritance, lack of enzymatic activity and dysfunction within DNA methylation cycles.
4. Having poor gut health can lead to an overabundance of bacterial strains that will promote production of free histamine.
5. Leaky gut/Intestinal Permeability can decrease the amount of Diamine Oxidase that is produced to properly break down histamine.
6. Stool and blood testing is VITALLY important to know what treatment will be needed to promote gut health.

7. Know what conditions and consumables may lead to an increase in the Histamine response and a decrease in Diamine Oxidase.

8. If you truly have a Histamine Intolerance, you must fix your digestive tract before you hope to limit the amount of systemic inflammation from the Histamine response.

Relationships: They Matter

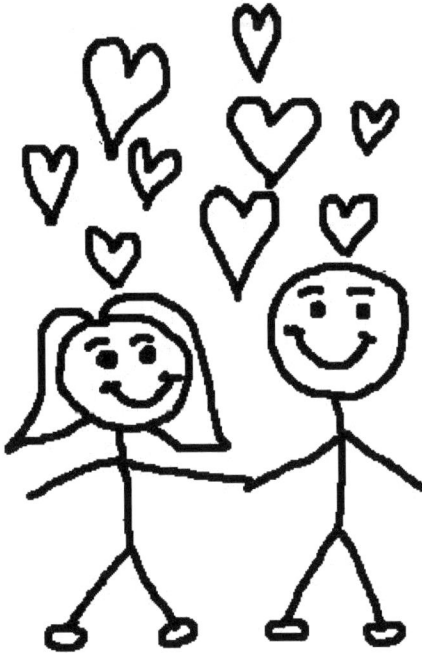

"The way we communicate with others and with ourselves ultimately determines the quality of our lives."
-Tony Robbins

Before you run away and think I am going to get into some wishy-washy lovey-dovey mumbo-jumbo, I want you to understand that the way you perceive the world is super relevant to how you perceive yourself. Confidence, determination, strong-willed, compassionate, loving, personable, marketable, vulnerable, teachable. To me that sounds like a human that anybody on Earth would like to be around. The reality is that these traits don't exist all at once. Humans weren't created to be a perfected, polished trophy that sits high upon a shelf for all to gaze upon. Because even beneath an immaculate trophy of prestige, honor and valor, there will always be imperfections. This is what makes us who we are. This is what makes us individuals. This is what makes us human.

The point I am driving at is simple. Accept yourself for who you are and who you will become. Never try to be like anyone else. Never think because of your eczema that you aren't good enough. Do not hide from your friends, family and the world to stave off embarrassment. I did this, and it added much more stress to my life and my personal relationships. Spend each day figuring out all of the qualities you possess. Figure out what makes you so different from everyone else and strive to set yourself further away from normal. Don't become part of the "in crowd." Make your own crowd! You and I are a part of each other's crowd and I welcome you to mine with open arms!

Christmas 2015 - I was going through the peak of my healing process. My brother was in from California to celebrate Christmas and ring in the new year with my family. During this time of the year, all of my best friends fly back into Tampa, FL to hang out and catch up for a week. We typically congregate at my friend Tommy's house. I remember passing his house on the way home and seeing all of my friend's cars parked in the driveway. I ducked my head as I snuck by quickly. During this week, my friends tried calling me, texting me and even Facebook messaging me to find out where I was. I screened every single one of their phone calls and text messages. I did not respond to a single one. The reason being: I was terrified to face my friends. I was scared of what they would think of me. I had weighed 145lbs soaking wet, down from 180lbs at 5'10. My eyes looked sunken in, skin in disarray and apathy was at an all-time high. They were going to engage in drinking and eating foods that I was not able to consume. So, I figured I would just avoid them at all cost. How disgustingly and incredibly selfish of me.

My friends, who dearly wanted to see me and who truly love me, were let down by my own decision to shut them out of my life. Instead of facing them head on and giving them the opportunity to console me during my self-loathing episodes, I put them into a state of consternation and suffering. My 15-year-long friendships that had been established through loyalty, camaraderie and connection had almost been severed by my own stupidity to turn off the world around me for my own sick benefit. By consciously avoiding them it created much more stress to my body, than if I were to take only 10 minutes of explaining my story. Instead, I lived an entire week in fear that my friends were going to find me. Stress is not good when it comes to clearing eczema away. Don't allow unnecessary stress in your life, it will only hinder your recovery. Believe me. I know.

These are the people I confide in when I am lost. These are the people who will travel miles to see me. These are the people who stick up for me during a debacle. These are the people who will love and care for me until the day I die. Yet, I decided they weren't what I needed in my life at the time. I only needed myself. The truth is, I needed them more than I ever had in my entire life. I love them. They are a part of me. They are my family.

Do not discount the power of community. When you are down in the dumps, or upset in any way, find someone who will listen to you. If your family or friends won't listen to you, find someone who will! There are always people willing to hear your story. I don't care who you are, everybody has a story that is worth sharing. Find online groups/forums, local community groups and even people like myself who just want to help. No matter what you are going through, just know someone has been in the exact same place you are currently in now. They too found guidance and help through community. They found the answer to their truest goals and desires. Emulate those who came before you. Adopt those core steps and concepts that paved the path for their success.

The story of Mrs. Jones

I want to tell you a quick story of a woman named Mrs. Jones. This was a patient of Dr. Goldberg's who came in with back pain that could not be explained by anything. X-rays and blood work all normal. He performed chiropractic adjustments multiple times, and nothing was relieving the discomfort. After a few months Mrs. Jones had not come in or made an appointment. Dr. Goldberg was getting worried, as Mrs. Jones was not in good health. One more month had passed by and Dr. Goldberg finally heard back from Mrs. Jones.

It turns out that when Mrs. Jones had been receiving care from Dr. Goldberg, she was severely depressed due to the death of her last husband. This depression was causing her intractable pain that Dr. Goldberg couldn't figure out.

However, for the months that Mrs. Jones had been missing in action, she had fallen madly in love with a new man. She reported that the day she met her new companion that all the pain in her body escaped her. She had never felt more alive.

Her pain was driven by the deep feeling of isolation and loneliness. Her emotions were so strong that they were directly impacting her physiology. This goes to show how POWERFUL human connection, companionship and relationships are.

Everyone deserves to be loved. To be cared for. To be listened to. Surround yourself by those who cherish your presence, your inner beauty and your heart.

Relationships recap:
1. Always remember that nobody is born a golden child. Everyone on Earth has their flaws even if they seem perfect. You will always be you. Figure out how to enhance what you already have!
2. Don't feel embarrassed by your skin. It is only a phase in your life. It is a struggle that will make you more powerful than anyone else. Don't feel like you must join a crowd to fit in. Create your own following!
3. Do not do what I did. Don't alienate your friends and family for fear that they will judge you. They are your friends for a reason. They love you! They will always be there for you. The more time you spend in fear without asking for help, the more stress you will endure by hiding from reality. Eczema will get worse.
4. Find and seek community. There will always be someone that will hear your story. Groups and communities are created each day for those who suffer will specific ailments. Never be scared to ask for help. People have been there before, and they know what works.

You Decide Your Health. End of Story.

You see, there are ONLY TWO directions in life:
You are either moving backwards into DISEASE or you are moving forwards towards HEALTH.

You will need to be the person who makes that decision.
Not me. Not your mom or dad. Not your dog. Not your siblings.

YOU.

You must realize, you get to choose how long and how well you want to live in this life.
Either pay THOUSANDS in medical bills, doctor's appointments, prescription medications now and later

OR

Make an investment in your health NOW to live LONGER, STRONGER and SMARTER with an abundance of VITALITY and HAPPINESS.

You can only be so successful in your family life, business life and personal life until you realize disease has you by the horns and it is way too late.

By taking the INVESTMENT in your health NOW, you make a MASSIVE investment in your potential productivity by having CRYSTAL CLEAR mental focus, an UNSHAKEABLE emotional state, ELATION every waking second, PEAK physical performance and UNPARALLELED personal relationships.

This life we live comes at a cost that YOU get to decide EVERY SINGLE DAY.

I can guide you to the promise land, the big show, the oasis and the gates of ultimate reward:

IT IS YOU that must make the decision to have a clear mind, open heart and OVERWHELMING desire to become:

MORE THAN YOU WERE YESTERDAY.
MORE THAN YOU EVER WILL BE
MORE THAN JUST ECZEMA FREE.
MORE THAN HUMAN...

AN **UNLEASHED** HUMAN

Setting The Stage For The Unleashed Human Lifestyle:

The beginning of this program is DESIGNED to DECREASE systemic inflammation and reset your digestive tract.

Once this SHORT phase is over, you will graduate into a full on UNLEASHED HUMAN:

Following the Unleashed Food choices composed of grass-fed, pasture-raised, wild-caught meats and organic produce and food.

Food guidelines are also to be supplemented with a healthy, physical, personal and mental lifestyle habits that come full circle.

You see – The Unleashed Human is much more than being Eczema Free:

It's a way of life. A way to be set free. A way to become EXTRA-ordinary.

Break the chains. Cut the ties. Burn the boats. Harness Unlimited Power. UNLEASH the beast.

Your Metamorphous Begins Here:
Your Most Ultimate Transformation

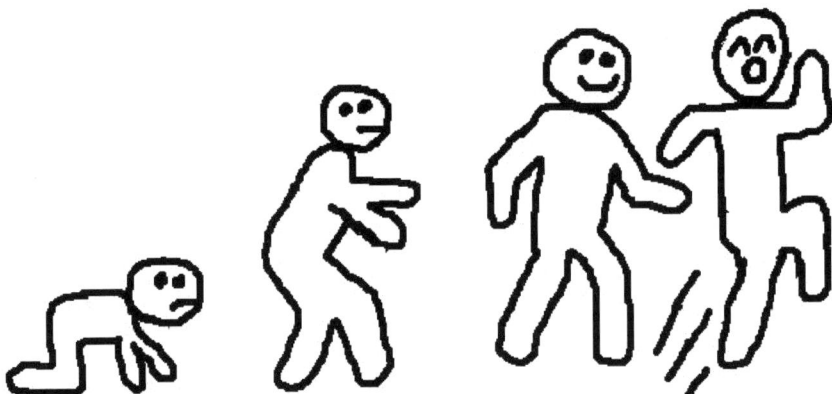

"You're always one decision away from a totally different life."
-Anonymous

"It's not about perfect. It's about effort. And when you implement that effort into your life. Every single day, that's where transformation happens. That's how change occurs. Keep going. Remember why you started."
-Anonymous

Week 1: (Days 1-7)

Morning
1. Open blinds, let sunshine in.
2. Make up your bed.
3. Walk outside to greet the morning and gather your thoughts.
4. Journal to your heart's desire.
5. Begin morning priming and breathing drills.
6. Go kick today's ass.
7. Drink 8oz glass of water without rice protein.
8. Prepare another 8oz glass of water with 2 scoops of rice protein.
9. Take multivitamin, vitamin C, and any other supplement I recommended specifically for you through coaching program.
10. If you prepared the vegetable broth, drink a glass.

Afternoon
1. Drink 8oz of water without rice protein.
2. Prepare another 8oz of water and mix with 2 scoops of rice protein.
3. Get 10-20 minutes of sunlight on both sides of body, making sure not to burn.
4. If you prepared the vegetable broth, drink a glass.

Night: Drink rice protein 3 hours before bedtime
1. Drink 8oz of water without rice protein.
2. Prepare another 8oz glass of water with 2 scoops of rice protein.
3. Take multivitamin, vitamin C, and any other supplement I recommended specifically for you through coaching program.
4. If you prepared the vegetable broth, drink a glass.
5. When the sun sets put on blue blocking glasses to stimulate melatonin release.

6. Complete your Journal entry for the day – what you did well, what you can make better.
7. In bed by 9pm, asleep by 10pm. (When you get there)

Week 2: (Days 8-15)

Morning
1. Open blinds, let sunshine in.
2. Make up your bed.
3. Walk outside to greet the morning and gather your thoughts.
4. Journal to your heart's desire.
5. Begin morning priming and breathing drills.
6. Go kick today's ass.
7. Drink 8oz glass of water without rice protein.
8. Prepare another 8oz glass of water with 2 scoops of rice protein.
9. Take multivitamin, vitamin C, and any other supplement I recommended specifically for you through coaching program.
10. If you prepared it, drink a glass of vegetable broth.

Afternoon:
1. Drink 8oz of water without rice protein.
2. Prepare another 8oz of water and mix with 2 scoops of rice protein.
3. You may have salad greens, non-starchy vegetables with oils/spices that are on the allowable list.
4. If you prepared it, drink a glass of vegetable broth.
5. Get 10-20 minutes of sunlight on both sides of body, making sure not to burn.

Night: Eat food and drink rice protein 3 hours before bedtime
1. Drink 8oz of water without rice protein.
2. Prepare another 8oz glass of water with 2 scoops of rice protein.

3. Take multivitamin, vitamin C, and any other supplement I recommended specifically for you.
4. You may have salad greens, non-starchy vegetables with oils/spices that are on the allowable list.
5. If you prepared it, drink a glass of vegetable broth.
6. When the sun sets put on blue blocking glasses to stimulate melatonin production.
7. Complete your Journal entry for the day – what you did well, what you can make better.
8. In bed by 9pm, asleep by 10pm. (When you get there)

Week 3: (Days 16-23)

Morning
1. Open blinds, let sunshine in.
2. Make up your bed.
3. Walk outside to greet the morning and gather your thoughts.
4. Journal to your heart's desire.
5. Begin morning priming and breathing drills.
6. Go kick today's ass.
7. Drink 8oz glass of water without rice protein
8. Prepare another 8oz glass of water with 2 scoops of rice protein.
9. Take multivitamin, vitamin C, and any other supplement I recommended specifically for you through coaching program.
10. If you prepared it, drink a glass of vegetable broth.
11. If you KNOW that you don't have an allergy to nuts or seeds, you may have walnuts, pistachios, macadamia and pecans.

Afternoon
1. Drink 8oz of water without rice protein.
2. Prepare another 8oz of water and mix with 2 scoops of rice protein.
3. You may have salad greens, non-starchy vegetables with oils/spices that are on the allowable list.

4. If you prepared it, drink a glass of vegetable broth.
5. Get 10-20 minutes of sunlight on both sides of body, making sure not to burn.
6. If you KNOW that you don't have an allergy to nuts or seeds, you may have walnuts, pistachios, macadamia and pecans.

Night: Eat food and drink rice protein 3 hours before bedtime
1. Drink 8oz of water without rice protein.
2. Prepare another 8oz glass of water with 2 scoops of rice protein.
3. Take multivitamin, vitamin C, and any other supplement I recommended specifically for you.
4. You may have salad greens, non-starchy vegetables with oils/spices that are on the allowable list.
5. If you prepared it, drink a glass of vegetable broth,
6. When the sun sets put on blue blocking glasses to stimulate melatonin production.
7. Complete your Journal entry for the day – what you did well, what you can make better.
8. In bed by 9pm, asleep by 10pm. (When you get there)

Week 4: (Days 24-31)

Morning
1. Open blinds, let sunshine in.
2. Make up your bed.
3. Walk outside to greet the morning and gather your thoughts.
4. Journal to your heart's desire,
5. Begin morning priming and breathing drills.
6. Go kick today's ass.
7. Drink 8oz glass of water without rice protein.
8. Prepare another 8oz glass of water with 2 scoops of rice protein.
9. Take multivitamin, vitamin C, and any other supplement I recommended specifically for you through coaching program.

10. If you KNOW that you don't have an allergy to nuts or seeds, you may have walnuts, pistachios, macadamia and pecans.

Afternoon
1. Drink 8oz of water without rice protein.
2. Prepare another 8oz of water and mix with 2 scoops of rice protein.
3. You may bake wild caught fish, salad greens, non-starchy vegetables with oils/spices that are on the allowable list.
4. If you KNOW that you don't have an allergy to nuts or seeds, you may have walnuts, pistachios, macadamia and pecans.
5. Get 10-20minutes of sunlight on both sides of body, making sure not to burn.

Night: Eat food and drink rice protein 3 hours before bedtime
1. Drink 8oz of water without rice protein.
2. Prepare another 8oz glass of water with 2 scoops of rice protein.
3. Take multivitamin, vitamin C, and any other supplement I recommended specifically for you through coaching program.
4. You may bake wild caught fish, salad greens, non-starchy vegetables with oils/spices that are on the allowable list.
5. When the sun sets put on blue blocking glasses to stimulate melatonin production.
6. Complete your Journal entry for the day – what you did well, what you can make better.
7. In bed by 9pm, asleep by 10pm. (When you get there).

Weeks 5-8:
Follow all steps for week 4 to let the stomach rest just a little longer

Weeks 9-12:
Follow all steps for week 4
Add in organic grass-fed beef and organic turkey/chicken if desired.
Try to only have 1 serving of meat source per day.

For those who did not purchase the Unleash Human Rice Protein:

1. You can either purchase it on my website: www.theunleashedhuman.com/riceprotein

   OR

2. You can choose to do a strict **vegetable ONLY** nutrition plan for 60 days:

1st Week Will ONLY consist of:
ORGANIC mixed salad greens with olive oil and minimal salt
THAT IS IT!

This week will not be easy. It will be tough. Without struggle, you will not be able to relish in victory. Just remember what the bigger goal is. In order to eliminate your eczema, you must allow your stomach to rest and re-cooperate from all of the years of damage. It is only seven days long! You've got this!

2nd week through 8th week: will ONLY consist of:
Non-starchy vegetables that were previously listed.
They MUST be steamed and making sure NOT to burn or char them!
You may add coconut oil or olive oil to them with minimal salt.

9th-10th week: YOU MUST MAKE SURE TO CHEW YOUR FOOD TO A PULP!!!

Remember – you have only been eating vegetables for the past 8 weeks. You have not been exposed to animal proteins in a long time. These proteins are much harder to break down than plant proteins and can be overwhelming for your body. Make sure to chew slow and chew well to help your digestion ease back into eating meats!

You may start adding in WILD-caught Salmon or Mahi.
You will want to bake your fish and not cook on grill or pan.
Make sure to continue to eat your vegetables!
You want your plate to be 20% meat (size of your fist) and 80% vegetables.

11th week and onward - You may start implementing:
ORGANIC - Pasture-raised chicken and grass-fed beef.

Notice: Your healing process may take a bit longer if you decide to go without the rice protein. Everyone is different and healing times **CAN VARY.** HOWEVER, if you follow the guidelines of this book STEP BY STEP, your chances of eliminating your eczema are HIGH.

IF YOU HAVE ANY PRE-EXISTING AUTOIMMUNE DISEASE OR CONDITION THAT IS SERIOUS ENOUGH TO BE ON MULTIPLE MEDICATIONS PLEASE DO NOT START THIS PLAN WITHOUT FIRST CONSULTING YOUR CURRENT MEDICAL DOCTOR.

PLEASE BE ADVISED: IF YOU HAVE OR HAD ANY HISTORY OF CANCER, PLEASE CHECK WITH YOUR MEDICAL DOCTOR OR SPECIALIST BEFORE ATTEMPTING ANYTHING I RECOMMEND HERE.

IF YOU ARE SICK OF WHAT YOUR MEDICAL DOCTOR HAS TO SAY AND WANT TO SCHEDULE A ONE-ON-ONE CONSULT WITH ME TO DISCUSS YOUR OPTIONS, BY ALL MEANS, PLEASE REACH OUT TO ME.

<u>AGAIN:</u> PLEASE DO NOT ATTEMPT OR CONTINUE THIS PLAN IF YOU HAVE A SERIOUS MEDICAL CONDITION IN WHICH YOU ARE NOT FIT TO TAKE A RADICAL CHANGE IN YOUR CURRENT STATE.

Foods Allowed:

Always try to buy organic foods and vegetables whenever possible.
Vegetables must be steamed. Never eat vegetables raw and do not
burn vegetables with char.

Vegetables:
Mixed greens
Carrots
Cucumber
Radishes
Kale
Collard greens
Brussel sprouts
Asparagus
Zucchini squash

Meats:
Wild caught baked Salmon or Mahi (allowed at 4th week)
Grass-fed or Organic Beef (to be consumed later in the program)
Organic Chicken or Turkey (to be consumed later in the program)
Pasture Raised/Organic WHOLE eggs (to be consumed later if you
have no allergy to eggs)

Oils/Spices:
Cold-pressed olive oil and coconut oil
Himalayan sea salt

Liquids:
Water
Homemade vegetable broth

Nuts/Seeds (allowed at week 3 if you know your nuts allergies):
Pistachio
Walnuts
Pecans
Macadamia

Foods Not Allowed:

Vegetables:
White potatoes, sweet potatoes, yams, and anything else related to a potato
Corn and corn products of any kind
Peppers, tomatoes, eggplant, onion, pumpkin, tapioca, starches, mushrooms

Legumes:
Beans of any kind (black, pinto, red, lima, green, chickpeas, peas, soybeans)
Peanuts, peanut butter, lentils, soy products (these should never be eaten)

Nuts/Seeds:
Sunflower seeds, sesame seeds, almonds, cashews, pine nuts, hazelnuts

Additives/Sweeteners:
No sugar, sweeteners of any kind, honey, molasses, maple syrup

Liquids:
No soda or juices (EVER)
No beer, wine, liquor or alcohol of any kind

Dairy (never allowed):
Milk, butter, cheese, cream cheese, whipped cream, half and half and anything milk related

Fermented foods
No kombucha, kefir, kimchi, sauerkraut or fermented foods of any kind

Wheat:
No breads or grains containing gluten

Meats:
No shellfish, pork, eggs, smoked meats, shrimp, tuna (too much mercury), tilapia, catfish

Oils/Spices/Dressings
Hot sauce, ketchup, tomato sauce, tomato products, paprika, black pepper, salad dressings
Canola oil, corn oil, cottonseed oil, grapeseed oil, peanut oil, safflower oil, sunflower oil

Food, Life and Mindset Going Forward

Your eating routine moving forward should be centered around clean organic vegetables and responsibly sourced, organic, wild caught and pasture-raised meats. This resembles and emulates the way we ate when we grazed off the land. Past the three-month mark of your meal plan, you will want to continue this routine and adopt it as your new way of eating. I never like to classify the way I eat into a category or diet fad. However, if you were to categorize it as anything it would be a Ketogenic/Paleo lifestyle. I cringe when people say they are doing paleo and find out they aren't even doing it correctly. Paleo is one of the most overused and played out diets in recent years. The plan I provided for you is not intended to ever be considered a diet by any means. I am simply providing you the tools to reset your digestive tract. The beginning phases of this meal plan (weeks 1-4) are not to be continued long term. The only purpose of this phase, as I just mentioned, is to let your digestion reset itself so you can flush the built-up toxins and begin eating clean organic food choices. Again, this is NOT a detox.

One of my greatest mentors, Dr. Paul Goldberg, is the person who gave me the opportunity to find my health again. One thing he taught me was, "Diet is merely what you consume or put into your mouth. Diet itself, is only one part of nutrition." Dr. Herbert Shelton who was Dr. Goldberg's mentor established a profound definition of nutrition. "The sum total of all the processes and functions by which growth, development, maintenance and repair of the body and by which reproduction is accomplished." This means diet is not the only thing that will aid in your journey to excellent health. It must be an entire lifestyle approach as I have laid out for you.

Remember how important your mindset is. Remember to feed your headspace all that it deserves. After all, our brain is the one which controls our final actions. If your mind has never ending thunderstorms, nothing good will come of your life. Seek connection. Seek camaraderie. Seek community. Seek a life full of love. Seek those who care for you unconditionally. Know that you are in control of your own happiness. Your state of emotion forms from your own desire to create moments of pure elation. Surround yourself by those who always want to better themselves. Average, subpar, settling and getting by. Take these words and blow them into a trillion pieces. Never become defined by your ability to accomplish things without pushing past the boundaries of your capability. Growth must present discomfort to exist. Put yourself on full blast for the world to see. You are no longer part of anyone's world except your own.

It is your life. It is your time. It is your world. Live it **UNLEASHED.**

-Dr. T.J. Woodham

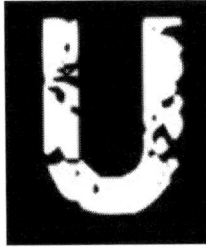

The Unleashed
EXPERIENCE:

As you may have read earlier, I do have an Unleashed Coaching Experience that allows you to have FULL access to me. This includes comprehensive lab tests, bonus health hacks, member gifts and exclusive recurring monthly content. Lab testing will be COMPLETELY and INDIVIDUALLY tailored based off an hour consultation. This will allow me to get to know you as an individual with a lifestyle plan SPECIFICALLY formulated for your needs. It also allows me to connect with you and create a lasting relationship experience.

My goal for you in this EXPERIENCE is to have your own health revelation and to teach the world a thing or two about health ;) I want you to become an empowered individual who cares about your health and the health of your loved ones. Everyone deserves to have a happy, long and healthy life. If I am able to create a chain reaction through my message so that you can help someone in desperate need for lifestyle modification, this will make me so happy. I want you to become more than you ever imagined was possible. For I am here at YOUR service.

I went through eight years of professional schooling and THOUSANDS of hours of personal research and development to give you all that I know. The good news for you is that... I never stop the hunger for learning, so as a member of my Unleashed Experience, you will get front row tickets to all the new content and knowledge I pump out every month!

However, this program is NOT for everyone. I DO NOT accept everyone who applies. Yes, there is an application you must fill out before I can start building a relationship with you. I don't mean this in a disrespectful or rude manner. Just like any relationship, we must be in mutual agreement that you will work hard, commit to the guidelines and go all in to become all you can be.

The Unleashed Experience is me serving YOU and HUMANITY on the highest level possible. I suffered by the clutches of eczema. I suffered the embarrassment and ridicule. I suffered the discomfort of oozing and itchy blisters. I suffered from the hiding from my family and friends. I've been through it all. It is about giving my knowledge and experience to those who still suffer. It would be selfish for me to keep all that I know about gaining clear skin, amazing digestion and incredible life habits from you.

If you are serious about making a commitment to yourself and to your health, please do yourself a favor and take that last leap of faith. It might just be the last best decision you make for your life, your health and your relationships.

BECOME.... **UNLEASHED**

Contact/Social Media

Join our members only Facebook group:
The Unleashed Human

Instagram:
@theunleashedhuman

Website:
theunleashedhuman.com

Connect with me for coaching inquiries:
theunleashedhuman@gmail.com

Bonus: 3 Simple Recipes

Recipe 1: Sunny Side Up Eggs with Carrots

Ingredients:

Pasture Raised Chicken Eggs
Himalayan Sea Salt
Organic Coconut oil
Organic Thyme
Organic Rosemary
Organic Carrots

Steps

1. Chop up 2 large carrots into thumb sizes pieces
2. Place the carrots into an Aroma Steam Cooker
3. Turn steam timer on to 10-12 minutes
4. Once carrots are done, add salt and either coconut oil or olive oil for greater taste

1. Grab medium frying pan and put coconut oil into the pan
2. Turn the burner on at medium heat (level 4-5)
3. Once oil starts to run, crack 4 eggs into the pan making sure they are spaced evenly
4. Place a lid over the pan and let them cook for 4-5 minutes
5. You will know the eggs are done when you start to see a white coating over the top of the yolk.
6. When done, add thyme, rosemary and salt

Eat and enjoy!

Recipe 2: Pork Chops and Broccoli

Ingredients:

Farm Fresh Pork chops
Himalayan sea salt
Organic Coconut Oil
Organic Thyme
Organic Rosemary
Organic Broccoli

Steps:

1. Cut organic broccoli florets off the stem or pre-chopped and place them into an Aroma Steam Cooker
2. Set the steam time to 12-14 minutes
3. Once done, add salt and either coconut or olive oil to give it better palatability.

1. Wash pork chops under water and then pat dry
2. Add thyme, rosemary and Himalayan salt to chops on both sides

1. Pre-heat oven to 360 degrees Fahrenheit
2. Grab baking pan and place tin foil inside of it
3. Spread coconut oil onto the foil evenly
4. Place the pork chops in the pain
5. When the oven is pre-heated, put the chops in the oven
6. Cook on one side for 15 minutes
7. After 15 minutes flip the chops onto the other side and then cook for an additional 15 minutes.
8. After the last 15 minutes, let the pork chop rest and cool.

Eat up and enjoy!

Recipe 3: Venison Steak

Ingredients:

Wild Game Venison
Himalayan Sea Salt
Organic Coconut oil
Organic Thyme
Organic Rosemary

Steps

1. Wash steak under water and then pat dry
2. Cut steak into thinner strips
3. Add thyme, rosemary and Himalayan salt to each strip on both sides
4. Grab medium frying pan and add coconut oil into the pan
5. Turn the burner on at medium heat (level 4-5)
6. Once oil starts to run, place the venison strips in the pain
7. Place a cover over the pan and let it cook for 5 min
8. After 5 min, flip the strips onto the other side and let cook for 2-3 minutes with lid on top.
9. After 2-3 minutes, the steak should be done.
10. Push it off to the side and let the steak rest, as it will continue to cook even off the burner

I didn't add vegetables for this recipe, but you can choose to follow the recipes I gave above or use the other vegetable recipes I have coming out soon.

These recipes are SUPER easy, and I did that for a reason.

We make the idea of cooking food and eating food this big ordeal and super complicated. We need to stop adding unnecessary ingredients and condiments to our foods.

Stick to the basics! It will cut down on time and money. Just get the absolutely important ingredients for your foods! Email me at theunleashedhuman@gmail.com if you would like the private links to these videos!

16414623R00079

Printed in Great Britain
by Amazon